"Chronic stress is a marker of living life on autopilot. This book gently wakes you up. It asks you instead to live life inside non-judgmental awareness and intentionality—and to do it right here, right now, in this moment. Written in Kirk Strosahl and Patricia Robinson's usual clear, step-by-step style, it contains scores of practical tips and exercises that gently train and practice a mindful path through stress. You cannot help but be moved."

> —**Steven C. Hayes, PhD,** cofounder of acceptance and commitment therapy (ACT) and author of *Get Out of Your Mind and Into Your Life*

in
this
moment.

FIVE STEPS *to*
TRANSCENDING STRESS
USING MINDFULNESS
and **NEUROSCIENCE**

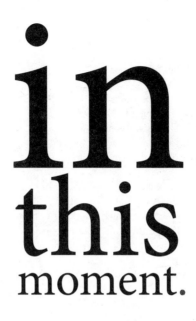

KIRK D. STROSAHL, PhD
PATRICIA J. ROBINSON, PhD

New Harbinger Publications, Inc.

Publisher's Note

Distributed in Canada by Raincoast Books

Copyright © 2015 by Kirk D. Strosahl and Patricia J. Robinson
 New Harbinger Publications, Inc.
 5674 Shattuck Avenue
 Oakland, CA 94609
 www.newharbinger.com

Self-assessments in chapter 3 of this book are adapted from the Five-Facet Mindfulness Questionnaire (FFMQ) in R. A. Baer, G. T. Smith, J. Hopkins, J. Krietemeyer, and L. Toney. 2006. "Using Self-Report Assessment Methods to Explore Facets of Mindfulness." Assessment 13:27–45. Used by permission of the authors.

Cover design by Amy Shoup
Acquired by Catharine Meyers
Edited by Jasmine Star

Library of Congress Cataloging-in-Publication Data

Strosahl, Kirk, 1950-
  In this moment : five steps to transcending stress using mindfulness and neuroscience / Kirk D. Strosahl and Patricia J. Robinson.
      pages cm
  Summary: "Little daily hassles can often add up to big stress. In In This Moment, two internationally-renowned psychologists show readers how to connect with the present moment and find a sense of calm and serenity using a breakthrough, evidence-based program grounded in mindfulness and neuroscience. Over time, chronic stress can take its toll on mental and physical health, leading to everything from anxiety and depression to weight gain and disease. By practicing the exercises in this book, readers will learn to combat stress in healthy ways, stay balanced, and live happier lives, no matter what challenges arise"-- Provided by publisher. *5544 0886 01/15*
  Includes bibliographical references.
  ISBN 978-1-62625-127-4 (paperback) -- ISBN 978-1-62625-128-1 (pdf e-book) -- ISBN 978-1-62625-129-8 (epub) 1. Stress management. 2. Meditation--Therapeutic use. 3. Neuroplasticity. 4. Neurosciences. I. Robinson, Patricia J. II. Title.
  RA785.S785 2015
  613--dc23
                                        2014033245

Printed in the United States of America

17   16   15

10   9   8   7   6   5   4   3   2   1   First printing

To my better half, Patti. How fortunate I am to have
you as my life partner and my writing partner!

—Kirk D. Strosahl

To Kirk, Lori, Donna, Pam, Judy, Regan Lara, Joanna May, Frances
Ann, and the other 7.046 billion kindred spirits on planet Earth;
my prayer in this moment is that you respond mindfully to stress.

—Patricia J. Robinson

Contents

Introduction

Stress researchers used to believe that the impact of big life events, such as divorce, natural catastrophes, or the death of a loved one, were the biggest threats to our health and well-being. Then they discovered that the real threat to emotional and physical health is the day in, day out stress of living in modern society. Indeed, the pace of modern life seems to be accelerating ever more quickly, as one innovation after another is introduced to create "efficiency" in our daily routines, from how we communicate with one another to how work is done on an assembly line. We believe these changes are adding to, not easing, the problem of daily stress.

As people get more efficient, they tend to just add more things to their to-do lists, rather than devoting the time saved to leisure pursuits and relaxation. The clients we work with continue to complain about the same high stress levels we were hearing about one or two decades ago.

As it turns out, you don't have to be a victim of major life events to have your health permanently affected by stress. The daily hassles of modern life can do the job very nicely. Stress-related diseases like hypertension, cardiovascular disease, diabetes, and cancer are at all-time highs, and nearly 50 percent of people over age sixty have at least one chronic disease that directly results from and is made worse by stress (CDC 2009).

Many risk factors for developing chronic disease are often simply ill-fated attempts to cope with daily stress. Eating can reduce stress but may also lead to obesity. Smoking is relaxing but leads to heart disease and cancer. Mental and social health are also directly affected by stress, with daily stress having been linked to problems with depression, anxiety, and anger, to name a few. Stress affects relationships with partners, children, family, friends, coworkers, and others. In general, it seems that most people have a very limited tool kit for dealing with the daily stress of life and could benefit from learning a few more tricks.

The Benefits of a Mindfulness-Based Lifestyle

This book is driven by our desire to promote a new approach to contemporary living and the stress it produces. We believe that adopting a mindfulness-based lifestyle allows people to be in the present moment, experience the joy of being alive, and act with a sense of life purpose.

Why would mindfulness act as a protective factor against the ravages of daily stress? The short answer is that, when uncontrolled, stress-related physiological arousal creates toxic neurochemical reactions in the brain and internal organs that can damage both physical and mental health. Mindfulness strategies activate portions of the nervous system that function to offset and control the harmful physiological effects of stress.

The better you get at using mindfulness strategies in your daily routine, the more able you'll be to regulate the noxious impacts of stress. Apart from this important benefit, practicing mindfulness in daily life can produce positive changes in mental outlook, improve social health, and increase mental efficiency. The skills taught in this book are based in cutting-edge research into the core facets of mindfulness. It turns out that mindfulness is not just one skill; it's a collection of unique abilities, each of which is important for creating a stress-transcending lifestyle.

As with any lifestyle change, bringing mindfulness to daily living involves a commitment to practice, even if for just a few minutes each day, mental or physical behaviors that bring you into direct contact with life on life's terms. Fortunately, practicing mindfulness strategies on a regular basis actually strengthens neural networks in the brain, making it increasingly easy to be mindful in times of stress. If you make the same commitment to training your brain that you make to exercising your body, you can experience powerful benefits, and you can experience them immediately. This is good news indeed, as many of these benefits, particularly positive mental health, healthy relationships, and improved cognitive efficiency, were previously thought to accrue only after years of daily meditation or mindfulness practice.

Neuroscience and Mindfulness

There has been explosion of interest in understanding how to integrate concepts in neuroscience and mindfulness to promote better physical and psychological health (Hanson 2011; Hanson and Mendius 2009). Contrary to earlier tenets of neuroscience, we now know that the brain is a dynamic organ that can alter the strength of its neural circuits to adapt to the demands of the immediate environment, a phenomenon known as *neuroplasticity*.

The main implication of neuroplasticity is that, with training, the brain can perform new functions or strengthen its existing functions. Research indicates that brain training involving mindfulness practices can strengthen areas of the brain responsible for attention, emotional control, and problem solving (Tang et al. 2007; Schuyler et al. 2012). (Indeed, if you search the Internet for brain training programs, you'll probably be surprised at the number, scope, and sophistication of products available to the general public.) At this point, it's clear that the routines people practice in daily life directly strengthen the underlying neural networks that support those routines (Slagter, Davidson, and Lutz 2011). There is even emerging evidence that mindfulness-based brain training produces permanent structural changes in the brain (Hölzel et al. 2011).

About This Book

This book is written to explain the relationship between stress, mindfulness, and neuroscience in as simple a way as possible. Therefore, we've made a dedicated effort to reduce the use of technical terms. We've also organized the book so that it's simple and easy to follow.

In part 1, A New Perspective on Dealing with Daily Stress, there are three chapters designed to help you get your feet on the ground, assess where you are right now, and create your learning plan. In chapter 1, we'll teach you more about daily stress and help you assess your current symptoms of daily stress. We'll also introduce the concept of mindfulness and link it to a neuroscience-based model of stress.

In chapter 2, we'll discuss the challenges of practicing mindfulness in the context of having a mind that doesn't necessarily want to cooperate! Your mind functions as a kind of internal advisor, and often its advice is for you to avoid, escape from, or ignore stress, rather than confront it in a healthy way. We'll explain how attempts to escape from or avoid dealing with stressful emotions are what actually activates the stress arousal system. Practicing mindfulness strategies will stimulate a different part of your nervous system—one that produces profound states of calm, detachment, and tranquility.

In chapter 3, we'll describe the five basic mental skills that collectively contribute to living mindfully. We'll help you assess your strengths and weaknesses in each of these five areas. You can then use the results of these self-assessments to create a skills development plan to guide your practice of mindfulness.

Part 2, Five Steps to Transcending Stress, has five chapters, each examining one of the five core aspects of mindfulness in detail: *observing, describing, detaching, loving yourself,* and *acting mindfully*. Each chapter includes a number of brain training exercises to help you strengthen the underlying neural circuitry of the brain that's responsible for that particular facet of mindfulness. These exercises are usually fun and quite brief and can be practiced on the fly as part of your daily routine. We also present a number of new mindfulness techniques, or practices, in each chapter. It's okay to pace your practice of these techniques as you work your way through the book; if a particular brain training exercise is new to you, continue to practice it until you feel you're pretty good at it, then move on to another exercise.

Part 3, Developing a Mindful Lifestyle, will help you design a mindfulness-based lifestyle and put it into practice. In chapter 9, you'll complete a more comprehensive assessment of daily stresses in your life and identify activities that help you recharge your batteries. We call the latter *daily helpers,* and they will be an important part of your stress balancing act. Chapter 10 invites you to identify ways you can engage in a daily regimen of self-restorative behaviors and offers some simple mindfulness techniques that you can integrate into your self-care routines. Chapter 11 will help you take a more mindful approach to work or school. It will also help you expand your definition of work so that you can put work or school stress in better perspective. We'll give you some practical mindfulness techniques that you can use before, during, and after work or school. Chapter 12 explores bringing more mindfulness to relationships—a key approach, given that positive social connections are so important in reducing the impact of daily stress. We'll give you a series of simple and fun mindfulness practices that can improve your connections with the people you care about.

Some of the exercises in this book invite you to write about your experience, whether keeping a record of daily hassles, exploring your reactions to stress, or drafting a plan to create a lifestyle that transcends stress. For some exercises, you'll find downloadable worksheets or other materials at http://www.newharbinger.com/31274. (See the back of this book for instructions on how to access them.) Alternatively, you can create your own versions of these forms. While working your way through this book, you may wish to keep a special journal for completing the exercises, and for writing any thoughts or ideas you have about what you learn.

An Invitation

When we first dreamed and schemed about writing this book, two main ideas stood out. First, we wanted to keep the concepts of mindfulness simple so as not to overwhelm you with a bunch of airy-fairy, new age stuff. Second, we wanted to give you practical, doable strategies that can fit the typical lifestyle in this day and age. We know that you don't have a lot of extra time on your hands, and that the stressful demands of daily living won't go away. Thus, the strategies we'll teach you are portable and don't require a lot of time. They're the kind of things you can do as part of your morning routine, while you're commuting, during a break at work or at home, during lunch hour (while leaving time for you to eat a nutritious lunch!), as part of an after-work wind-down routine, or as part of your bedtime routine.

One thing we do ask is that you be persistent. Just as you have to exercise on a somewhat regular basis to improve your physical fitness, you can expect the benefits of mindfulness strategies to increase as you practice them consistently. As we like to say, practice doesn't make perfect; practice makes *permanent!* We sincerely hope that you take us up on this invitation to revitalize your life and transcend daily stress in the process.

PART 1

A New Perspective on Dealing with Daily Stress

CHAPTER 1

Stress, Mindfulness, and Neuroscience

Reality is the leading cause of stress
amongst those in touch with it.

—Jane Wagner

Chances are you picked this book up because you're concerned about the amount of stress you're experiencing and want to do something about it. Congratulations on your decision to do something about stress in your life before it gets the better of you! Being stressed-out is a very unpleasant place to be. It affects all aspects of your health and well-being, including how your body functions (causing indigestion, head-aches, diarrhea, sleep difficulties, appetite loss, and a host of other problems); your emotional health (leading to moodiness, sadness, anxiety, and so on); your mental focus (resulting in loss of concentration, forgetfulness, or distractibility); and your relationships with others (due to irritability, withdrawing from others, isolating yourself, and the like).

If you're experiencing any of these symptoms of stress, we want to assure you that you are definitely not alone: A national survey conducted by the American Psychological Association (2010) found that seven in ten Americans suffer from physical symptoms due to stress, and 67 percent report that they experience high levels of daily stress.

The main culprits causing their stress will undoubtedly sound familiar to you: lack of money, housing costs, job instability, work pressure, the economy, relationship problems, personal health concerns, health problems of loved ones, and concerns about personal safety. At the same time, 60 percent of those surveyed reported that they didn't take care of themselves very well. Only one out of four people reported exercising regularly, and half of the people surveyed reported concerns about their physical health, along with a variety of unhealthy coping behaviors, such as overeating, skipping meals, or alcohol or drug abuse.

It's a commonly accepted fact that chronic stress is also associated with the development of physical illnesses such as hypertension (high blood pressure), heart attack, stroke, diabetes, and cancer (CDC 2009). What most people don't appreciate is that the psychological distress triggered by stress can be a much stronger factor in producing heart attacks, strokes, and other adverse cardiovascular events than the risk factors we so often hear about through the media, such as smoking, obesity, or lack of exercise (Hamer, Malloy, and Stamatakis 2008). To make matters worse, prolonged exposure to stress is associated with the development of mental health problems. For example, about 50 percent of the people surveyed reported recurrent problems with depression, anxiety attacks, worry, irritability, anger management issues, or sleep problems. Because unresolved stress can be harmful to your physical and mental health, we want to congratulate you for taking on this problem right now, before things get worse. We want to help you transcend stress and create a vital, purposeful life in the process!

In this book, you'll learn a practical and highly portable five-pronged approach to building a personal sanctuary from stress and its ongoing negative effects on your mental and physical health. Inside this sanctuary, you can be aware of the stress around you without being consumed by it. You can be aware of your emotions, thoughts, memories, or physical symptoms without having to struggle with them. You can love yourself for who you are, warts and all. You can connect with what matters to you in your life and act with a sense of a personal mission. As you read the concepts in this book and practice the skills we outline, consider this your quest to turn yourself from Velcro, where every little stress sticks to you, even when you try to fling it off, to Teflon, where stress just slides off you without any effort at all!

Daily Hassles: It's the Small Stuff That Gets You!

While it is true that big life events, such as divorce, bankruptcy, or the death of spouse, have a negative impact on health and mental well-being, it appears that the small daily stresses of everyday living exert an even greater influence in the long term (Holm and Holroyd 1992). In this book, we sometimes use the phrase "daily hassles" to describe this kind of daily stress. One long-term study of daily hassles showed that they had a direct negative impact on physical health problems nearly a decade later, particularly among people with high levels of stress (Piazza et al. 2013). Daily hassles function somewhat like the ancient Chinese practice of water torture: one drop of water on your head doesn't seem like much until you've spent days on end experiencing one drop of water at a time.

A key factor to consider is that dealing with daily hassles is really a *lifestyle* issue, and therefore antistress measures need to be a basic part of your daily routine. The good news is, you don't need to use heroic coping measures, as might be the case with a major life event. Instead, you need to have a reliable set of daily go-to strategies that help you transcend daily stress and recharge your batteries.

On the downside, because chronic daily stress isn't likely to go away, it can be very tempting to try to ignore it or minimize its impact. You might think about how good you have it compared to someone you know: "Oh, my stress isn't all that bad. Look at my neighbor Sam. He lost his son in Afghanistan. Now, that's real stress." In other words, people tend to turn a blind eye to daily stress, assuming that it's just a part of living and there's nothing they can do about it. Only when their health or mental health collapses do they take action, and by then it's often too late.

Over time, daily hassles wear you down and decrease your motivation to participate in life. You might start going through each day rather mindlessly, living life on autopilot and doing things by force of habit, rather than out of desire. It's also kind of like cruise control, where you just push a button and the car takes over some of the main functions of driving. This might work well on a long road trip, but it sure doesn't work as a strategy for living a vital, purposeful life. When you're just trying to get through the day, you're much more likely to skip activities that could promote your sense of vitality and being truly alive. For example, instead of going to the movies with your children, you might make an excuse and get your spouse to go with them. Then, when they're gone and you're home alone, you might just take a nap or watch a TV rerun in a mindless kind of way.

Exercise: Stress Observation Survey (Or SOS!)

Before we teach you more about our approach to stress, we'd like you to take this short survey. It will help you get a better idea about how much daily stress might be affecting you. These items reflect some of the typical daily experiences that result from stress and living on auto-pilot. Read each item and put a check by it if that item applies to you.

_____ I feel tapped out by the end of a typical day.

_____ I feel rushed even when I'm running on time.

_____ I have trouble doing things at a slower pace, even when I have the time.

_____ I tend to think about what's coming up in my day rather than being in the here and now.

_____ I often want to be left alone when I get home from work or school.

_____ I find myself sighing a lot during the day.

_____ My eyes often burn early in the day.

_____ I often forget to take breaks because of the pressure I'm under.

_____ I find it difficult to relax even when I have free time.

_____ When I have free time, I prefer activities that help me zone out.

_____ *I have trouble motivating myself to do things that are healthy for me.*

_____ *I feel exhausted by the end of the day much of the time.*

_____ *I feel like I'm always running behind.*

_____ *I feel like I'm always multitasking, even at home.*

_____ *I often find myself daydreaming when I'm with my partner or children.*

_____ *I tend to bring my work or school stress home with me.*

_____ *I often wake up at night and think about things that are stressing me out.*

_____ *I notice that I get impatient and irritable about little things.*

_____ *I often do things like household tasks without even thinking about them.*

_____ *I feel like taking time to relax means I'll just fall behind on some duty or responsibility.*

Do any of these items ring a bell for you? If so, it's likely that daily stresses are building up and impacting how you're functioning. Often, this effect is very subtle, and only becomes obvious when you take a minute to review how you're doing. We want to help you stop this process from snowballing to the point where stress damages your mental or physical health.

Exercise: Recording Daily Hassles and Helpers

Even at this early point in the book, it might be useful for you to begin thinking broadly about some of the daily hassles you face and record-

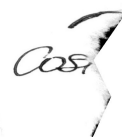

ing them. Right now, our main purpose is to get you thinkin-
this type of insidious stress and the specific forms it might to
you. Later, in chapter 9, we'll lead you through a comprehensive s-
assessment of these annoying, mood-damaging daily events.

As suggested earlier, you might also have some daily helpers.
go-to behaviors that help you recharge your batteries and offset the
draining effect of daily stress (Kanner et al. 1981). Start noticing and
listing your helpers now in a Daily Hassles and Helpers Log. Later, in
part 3 of the book, we'll guide you in creating a lifestyle plan in which
you deliberately balance daily hassles with daily helpers.

You'll find a downloadable worksheet you can use to record your
daily stresses and helpers at http://www.newharbinger.com/31274
(see the back of this book for instructions on how to access it). Alternatively, you can create a similar form, perhaps in your journal for this
book, using the three columns in the downloadable worksheet: "Day
of week and time" on the left, "Daily hassle" in the center, and "Daily
helper" on the right.

If you don't like to use tables or structured records, it's okay if you
simply make free-form notes. The main purpose of this exercise is to
help you start thinking about these issues in your life a little differently.
Later on, we'll use the information you've collected to develop a new
approach that will help you transcend stress.

Victims of Daily Stress

As practicing psychologists, we see firsthand the devastating effects of
stress on the lives of people who come to us seeking help. One of the
most notable aspects of the stories clients tell us about stress is how
ordinary life events, piled one on top of another, can end up creating
one stressed-out human being. Daily hassles are really sneaky. Taken
one at a time, they don't seem dangerous, but when they pile up on you,
significant problems can arise. The following true-life examples will
give you a glimpse of the huge variety of daily stressors out there and
how they can unravel a human life.

• Mary's Story

Mary fell victim to stress in her late twenties. She graduated from college on schedule, then broke up with her long-term boyfriend to pursue career opportunities and explore other options in relationships. The career ladder turned out to be very difficult to climb, requiring excessive work hours and too few financial incentives. Mary was particularly upset when she was passed over for a promotion that she thought she deserved. She experimented with going to happy hour with some coworkers and noticed that having a few drinks helped her relax and eased her bad attitude about her workplace. Soon she fell into a pattern of drinking at home after work, and before long, she started drinking most of the day on weekends. It wasn't until a close friend mentioned that her drinking seemed to be getting the best of her that Mary decided to do something about it.

She consulted an employee assistance program specialist at work, who taught her some deep breathing exercises and recommended that she practice them four to five times daily. The breathing strategies helped when she remembered to do them, but her long work hours and limited time for herself made regular practice difficult. Her counselor recommended that she set an alarm on her smartphone to remind her to practice. On several occasions the alarm went off while she was in the middle of a meeting at work and she couldn't excuse herself. After a while, being reminded to practice deep breathing annoyed her and made her even more anxious about the fact that she wasn't taking care of herself as she should. One day she turned the alarm off for good.

• Bob's Story

Bob began struggling with stress in his thirties. The company he worked for started experiencing financial problems; as a result, his workload increased, but his pay didn't. He was married and had two young children, and his wife was getting frustrated with him because she felt that the long hours Bob worked indicated that he was more committed to his job than to her and the kids. Bob couldn't see any way out of his situation, especially because his job was crucial for supporting his family. Over time, intimacy with his wife and interactions with his kids declined to the point that he was spending most of his time at home watching TV or surfing the Internet.

Bob started to experience more and more symptoms of depression, and he found that eating helped ease his depressed feelings, at least temporarily. Over a two-year period, Bob gained forty-five pounds and was eventually diagnosed with diabetes. He believed that his weight made him unattractive to his wife, so he avoided her even more. He also felt guilty for letting his health go and often forgot to monitor his blood sugar level.

Bob's physician asked him to start walking at least thirty minutes a day and recommended an Internet program that could track his daily calorie intake and walking. However, Bob had never been into exercise, and now his weight made walking physically uncomfortable. He also felt self-conscious and was sure that other people were judging him because of his weight. Still, he found a coworker he liked who was willing to walk with him every day during their lunch hour. They walked several times, but then Bob's department was assigned a new project that made it difficult for him to do anything other than, as he put it, "gobble, gulp, and go." Bob kept making excuses for not walking with his coworker, and eventually his coworker stopped asking.

• Linda's Story

Linda ran into problems with stress in her fifties after moving from her hometown to take care of her aging parents. Linda had always taken pride in her ability to keep her life in balance. She and her husband had always attended church, and her faith was an important part of her balancing act in life. After moving, Linda found a new job but not a new church. At her new job, she was earning less money despite working many more hours. In addition, she was cooking and cleaning for her parents several hours each day. She just didn't have as much time to practice her faith. When she had a few precious moments of free time, she usually turned on the TV and tuned out the world.

Over time, Linda started to resent her parents for "putting her" in such a stressful situation even though she knew it wasn't their fault. Her sister volunteered to come and take care of their parents for a couple of weeks, but Linda declined because her sister's husband was struggling with health issues and Linda didn't want to be responsible for creating even more problems for her sister. Linda went to her doctor because she was having trouble sleeping, and he prescribed an antidepressant, believing that her sleep problems might be a sign of depression. The medication helped her sleep better, but she felt more numbed out. There was no joy in her life, only the drudgery of daily duties.

The Problem: Avoiding Unpleasantness

We live in a culture that's obsessed with getting rid of any unpleasant physical or mental experiences, including the symptoms of daily stress. Our cultural definition of what it means to be healthy and happy includes being free of anything unpleasant or distressing. We're expected to have no skeletons in the closet. To help us achieve this idealized version of health and well-being, our culture has assembled an unprecedented arsenal of medications, supplements, and other remedies for anything that ails us, physically or emotionally. The problem is, the experience of being human includes having unpleasant, distressing reactions to the normal stresses of everyday existence.

Practically speaking, we've been taught to reject the growth-producing aspects of daily stress and instead focus our energy on finding ways to eliminate or control the symptoms of stress. Instead of seeing those symptoms as signals that life might be out of balance in some important way, we try to kill the messenger. For example, Bob's promotion triggered a variety of life changes that were for the worse, but rather than responding to his stress symptoms with helpful lifestyle changes, he started overeating to numb out his negative emotions. Instead of confronting his stress, Bob tried to avoid it, and it came back to bite him. Bob's story isn't unusual. We've all been taught to try to avoid or escape the pernicious effects of daily stress or numb ourselves to these effects. We do this mindlessly on a day in, day out basis.

The Solution: Mindfulness

As the title of this book suggests, we believe there's a better way to approach daily stress than giving in to it and living life on autopilot. This approach is called *mindfulness*. An easy-to-understand definition of mindfulness is that it involves "paying attention in a particular way: on purpose, in the present moment, and nonjudgmentally" (Kabat-Zinn 1994, 4). So one aspect of taking a mindful approach to stress is to pay attention to it, rather than trying to avoid, minimize, or ignore it. Mindfulness also means paying attention to stress in a particular way, remaining nonjudgmental about it and simply accepting the reactions it produces in you. This will give you a huge advantage, allowing you to think clearly about the actions you wish to take to offset the effects of stress.

Another extremely important aspect of taking a mindful approach to stress is learning to act with intention in the midst of stressful circumstances. With the clear mind that nonjudgmental attention creates, you can connect with what matters to you in life and choose actions that reflect what you care about. At the end of the day, you can even embrace daily stress as your teacher because it will give you a valuable opportunity to clarify what matters to you in life and organize your life accordingly. The only medicine we know of that can cure the problem of living life on autopilot is to live life deliberately, according to what matters to you.

When we ask you to embrace daily stress, we aren't saying you have to like living with stress. Rather, we're encouraging you to listen to your stress, accept that it's there, and adopt a deliberate, mindful approach that will help you transcend it. If you don't take a conscious, purposeful approach to the stress you're under, it will organize your life to its purposes. We often put it this way: if you aren't willing to have stress, then stress will have you.

Here's another thing to consider: the mere fact that you have daily stress means there are things in your life that you care about. If nothing mattered to you, you wouldn't have any stress at all. You're busy trying to accomplish something in your life—perhaps providing for your family, improving your job skills, or getting an education. There's nothing unhealthy about short-term stress reactions that arise in the context of these important life pursuits.

At the same time, living in a healthy way requires that you balance the stress you're under with a consciously constructed lifestyle that insulates you from the unhealthy, long-term effects of stress. This is hard to do if you're so busy avoiding the symptoms of stress that you can't turn your attention to the problem at hand. That's why we wrote this book: to help you learn, practice, and integrate skills that will allow you to live *with* stress, rather than trying to avoid it, pretend it isn't there, or numb yourself to its negative effects. At the end of this book, you'll be in a position to live a stress-transcending lifestyle and enjoy a full and rewarding life, even with the ongoing stress of having to adapt to life's changing circumstances.

The Neuroscience of Stress and Mindfulness

Fortunately, the emerging field of cognitive neuroscience is making it increasingly clear that you can train your brain to support you in taking a mindful approach to stress. With practice, you can achieve a more relaxed and transcendent state of mind that will override the rigid, anxious, autopilot mode that stress creates. Even better, the mental skills needed to make this shift aren't difficult to master, and they get stronger and stronger with practice.

In this section, we'll give you a brief lesson in brain anatomy and nervous system physiology so you can better understand how stress affects your brain and body. The brain consists of an elaborate system of neural circuitry that functions, in part, to help you maintain an ongoing balance between your stress and relaxation responses. This balancing act is achieved through continual interactions between two different parts of your nervous system: the reticular activating system and the dorsolateral prefrontal cortex.

The Limbic System

The *limbic system* is a complex set of brain structures that includes the hippocampus, hypothalamus, amygdala, and other nearby areas of the mammalian brain. It is primarily responsible for processing emotional responses to stress. The limbic system is integrated into an even more basic part of the nervous system: the *reticular activating system*.

The reticular activating system consists of the primitive part of the brain that produces emotional arousal and the well-known fight-or-flight response. This part of the brain evolved early on to offer protection from all kinds of natural threats to survival. Thus, it's exquisitely sensitive to any kind of threat—including threats we just imagine. So you can merely think of a stress-producing situation at work or school and trigger numerous physical, emotional, and mental stress reactions, even though you aren't actually in that situation. The branch of the nervous system that supports all of these stress-related changes is called the *sympathetic nervous system* (SNS). The name is ironic, because SNS activation makes you anything but sympathetic!

Sympathetic nervous system activation begins when some type of stress is detected that triggers the limbic system. Within a microsecond, the SNS initiates a cascade of changes in the body. Blood flow in the gut is directed instead to large muscle groups, to prepare them for immediate action, as well as areas in the mid-brain. The hypothalamic-pituitary-adrenal axis of your endocrine system works closely with the sympathetic nervous system and releases stress hormones, such as epi¬nephrine (adrenaline) and cortisol, into your bloodstream. These neu-rochemicals have an immediate impact on blood pressure, heart rate, and skin temperature. The release of cortisol, in particular, also creates cognitive confusion—which is why people under stress often complain of being confused and having difficulty accurately processing information and making decisions.

Unfortunately, even small daily stresses can stimulate the limbic system and produce powerful stress responses. This is why an awkward interaction with a coworker or classmate can be as stressful as having a tooth extracted. Chronic SNS arousal, a common result of ongoing daily stress, is also thought to be the underlying cause of most stress-related health illnesses, such as hypertension, heart disease, cancer, and diabetes.

The Dorsolateral Prefrontal Cortex

The second part of the brain that plays a key role in our response to stress is the *dorsolateral prefrontal cortex*. This region of the brain evolved later than the limbic system and is basically responsible for most of the higher-order functions we normally associate with being human: attention, emotion regulation, planning, abstract reasoning, and complex problem solving. This region of the brain is your friend when it comes to managing your response to stress. It's closely linked with the *parasympathetic nervous system* (PNS), a part of the brain that puts the brakes on all of the physical changes produced by the SNS. When your PNS is activated, your breathing rate and heart rate slow, your blood pressure decreases, and your blood supply is redirected to your brain.

The good news is that, although the effects of SNS activation are immediate and can seem overwhelmingly intense, in reality the PNS is much stronger. The SNS evolved to help us act quickly and effectively in response to a threat and then shut down once the danger has passed. The basic nature of the SNS is to shut down if it receives any type of signal to do so. Therefore, something as simple as taking one or two deep, slow breaths when you're under stress will immediately activate your PNS and help the SNS shut down. Better yet, applying the mindfulness techniques you'll learn in this book will help you counter immediate stress reactions and also produce states of relaxation and clarity of thought that are uniquely associated with prolonged activation of the PNS.

Guidelines for Brain Training

As we've mentioned, the brain is a dynamic organ that can be strengthened via mental exercise. So the question isn't whether the brain can be trained, but how best to train it. As it turns out, there's quite a bit of new, research-based information on this very topic. We want to share some of the more important findings because they'll provide guidance in creating your own brain training program and using that program to develop a mindful approach to daily hassles.

Your Undivided Attention Is Essential

As with creating any new brain habit, practicing mindfulness techniques requires that you pay attention to what you're doing. Research backs up this commonsense philosophy, with studies showing that the benefits for neural networks and brain structures only occur when people pay close attention while practicing a particular skill (Davidson and Begley 2012). In other words, learning to pay attention, which just happens to be the first skill needed to be in the here and now, is also necessary for any mental training to have an effect on your neural networks and brain structures. So if this approach is to be effective, you can't be half in the here and now while the other half of you is thinking about what you'll eat for dinner. You have to be willing to show up and pay close attention to the specific skill you're trying to master.

Vary What You Practice

Functional magnetic resonance imaging studies use highly sophisticated brain imaging technology to reveal the strength of electrical activation in certain areas of the brain produced while the subject is performing various mental tasks, such as paying attention, naming or responding to emotions, and observing physical sensations, to name but a few. The basic finding of interest is that the more regions of the brain that are activated by skill training, the stronger the overall effect is on brain efficiency (Davidson and Begley 2012).

For example, the benefits of practicing observing skills (which you'll learn in chapter 4) increase when you shift back and forth between what you're aware of externally—like objects, people, smells, or touch—and internally, like thoughts, feelings, or memories. The ability to observe external and internal information is controlled by different structures or neural networks in the brain, so repeatedly shifting focus on purpose strengthens the linkages between these seemingly distinct skills. Therefore, in this book we offer a variety of specific skills to practice; collectively, they'll give you a greater ability to activate your PNS.

Practice Produces Immediate Benefits

An earlier view of the brain was that it was relatively fixed and hard to rewire, which meant you might need to practice mindfulness for years before seeing any positive benefits. This made it difficult to sell mindfulness to the general public, given that most people are already overscheduled. Newer findings indicate otherwise, and one immediate implication of neuroplasticity is that changes in brain function can occur much more immediately.

One of the more astonishing findings in this respect comes from the cutting-edge work of neuroscientist Richard Davidson, at the University of Wisconsin. In one study, volunteers were taught a brief loving-kindness meditation in an attempt to compare the electrical patterns in their brains to those of experienced meditators. Remarkably, even after only minimal practice, novice meditators exhibited unique brain activity patterns that were nicknamed the "compassion wave" (Lutz et al. 2004). More recent results suggest that both emotional control and compassionate behavior toward the suffering of others are strengthened by even brief compassion meditation training (Lutz et al. 2008; Weng et al. 2013).

Practice Makes Permanent

Although brain changes can occur quickly, they aren't necessarily enduring. In the aforementioned study by Richard Davidson's team (Lutz et al. 2004), novice meditators did show almost immediate changes in brain readings, but their new patterns weren't as strong as similar patterns in the brains of experienced meditators. This suggests that extended practice does have benefits: the more you practice, the stronger your compassion wave gets. This type of finding is common in the brain training literature. The more you practice a specific mental skill, like paying attention, the more your brain circuitry evolves to support that skill. The increase in specific types of electrical activity among experienced meditators is probably the result of a far more integrated set of neural circuits and the direct result of prolonged daily practice. Again, to update the old saying, practice doesn't make perfect; practice makes permanent!

Throughout this book, we're going to emphasize that this is a lifestyle issue. You can't practice "drive-by" mindfulness and expect to benefit over the long haul. Then again, why would you want to? These are health-promoting, positive, prosocial skills that can play a huge role in helping you take a more balanced, compassionate approach to yourself and those you care about. Wouldn't you like to have even more empathy, love, and compassion than you already do? Wouldn't that be a good thing for you?

Use It or Lose It

A related finding is that, as with working out to build muscle, if you don't keep up your brain training regimen, new skills can begin to atrophy. In the University of Wisconsin studies (Lutz et al. 2004), the brain wave changes observed in novice meditators were astonishing but short-lived. Several weeks after the experiment concluded, a follow-up study was conducted to once again examine the brain wave patterns of the two groups of meditators, novice and experienced. Whereas the experienced meditators continued to exhibit the compassion wave at the same strength as before, novice meditators who had stopped practicing the compassion exercise no longer showed this change in their brain wave patterns. Therefore, ongoing practice of the techniques you learn in this book is important; otherwise you might begin slipping back into a stressed-out, autopilot mode. And this type of short-term neuroplasticity means that you're always training your brain to do something. If you don't pay attention to what you're doing, you could end up training your brain to stress you out!

Gentle Reminders

In this chapter, we introduced the idea that daily stress is a huge enemy in the quest to live the way you want to live. If you avoid, ignore, or downplay the importance of daily stresses, they can pile up and have a devastating impact on both your mood and your health. Therefore, we encourage you to take a more mindful approach to daily stress by paying attention to it and embracing it in a nonjudgmental way. This will help you think clearly about what matters to you in your life and then act intentionally, in ways that reflect your principles.

The tenets of neuroscience offer a fresh perspective on how you can train your brain to support a mindful approach to daily stress. You can directly train your brain to reduce the influence of harmful physiological and mental effects of stress while also increasing your ability to induce states of mindful awareness. But brain science isn't a panacea for problems with becoming present and following through with your mindfulness game plan. You'll have to commit to practicing new strategies and doing so persistently over time.

In our culture, we're bombarded by messages to exercise more often as a way to strengthen our bodies and prevent disease. Yet people often twist their faces in distaste when the discussion turns to the virtues of brain training. For most people, the prospect of coming into contact with their mind on a daily basis seems to be much more aversive than engaging in vigorous physical exercise. In the next chapter, we'll explore why this is. In large part, it happens because the mind doesn't necessarily want to cooperate!

CHAPTER 2

Mindfulness and the Art of Living with Your Mind

I used to think that the brain was the most wonderful
organ in my body. Then I realized who was telling me this.

—Emo Phillips

In chapter 1, we looked at the problem of daily stress from a different
perspective, closely linking the practice of mindfulness to improved
brain functioning and the ability to transcend stress. With practice,
you can train your brain to help you implement a more mindful
approach to the challenge of living with daily hassles. Of course, there
will be difficulties along the way. One problem is that people don't
relate directly to the brain. Instead, we interact with its end product:
the internal advisor often called the *mind*. Your mind may actually
advise you to use ineffective strategies for stress because it believes
you'll feel better if you simply avoid unpleasant emotions or physical
symptoms. There's even a saying that expresses this common point of
view: out of sight, out of mind. In all likelihood, your mind may not be
willing to cooperate with you as you attempt to deal with daily stress in
a more mindful way.

Thus, learning to be mindful requires more than just paying attention to daily stress in different ways. It also requires that you pay attention to the activities of your internal advisor in a different way. To help
you do this, we'll teach you to look at your mind a little differently than
you might be doing now. This new perspective will allow you to relate
to your mind in a different way when doing so is worthwhile. To develop

this new relationship with your mind, you first need to understand what the mind is, why it's sometimes problematic to have a mind, and how practicing mindfulness offsets some of the negative tendencies of the mind.

Finally, we'll introduce you to two radically different states of mind: restless mind and quiet mind. Restless mind is hardwired to keep you in a constant state of arousal and busyness, which amplifies the negative impacts of stress. Quiet mind allows you to be aware of the moment, experience a sense of peace and tranquility, feel compassion for yourself and others, and make direct contact with what matters to you in life. We're pretty sure that, if you could choose between the two, you'd pick the second one. Fortunately, learning to choose your state of mind is exactly what this book is designed to help you do!

Mind: The Brain's Operating System

People sometimes get confused when we talk about the mind and the brain as if they were two different things, but they are. First of all, the brain is a thing—a physical structure. You can see it on a functional magnetic resonance image. It has shape, weight, size, and texture. The electricity generated by neurons can be measured by an electroencephalograph. However, you never make direct contact with the biological activities of the brain. You don't hear the rumble of neurons firing or feel a slight shock as neurons exchange electrical charges, and you can't send orders to your midbrain telling it to calm down.

On the other hand, you *are* in contact with your brain's operating system: your mind. If you think of your brain as a supercomputer, then you can think of the mind as the computer operating system, like Windows or Mac OS X. The brain's operating system continually feeds you messages, not unlike words or images on a computer monitor. Often these messages come in the form of a silent inner dialogue; it's almost like interacting with an inner advisor. We humans use the inner advisor to interpret life experiences and their meaning, to solve daily problems both small and large, and to decipher emotions and take action. It would be fair to say we live in our minds.

The interaction between the mind and the brain is a two-way street. The brain delivers messages directly into the mind (for example, in the form of vision, hearing, smell, or pain), and the mind delivers messages directly to the brain. For example, you might hear a song that reminds you of a past relationship that ended very badly. Even though the song itself is beautiful to listen to, the message sent to your brain is that this is sad. The brain then triggers an emotional event in the reticular activating system, and you experience sadness while listening to the song. Indeed, brain training is based on the idea that you can capitalize on this basic relationship: that you can use your mind to train your brain to support mindfulness processes in your everyday life (Hanson and Mendius 2009).

The Nature of the Mind

It's no accident that the world's religious and meditative traditions have focused, in one way or another, on trying to understand the nature of the mind so we can be better equipped to deal with it. We're so used to contacting the mind that we forget it isn't good at everything. Yes, it knows how to help you balance a checkbook, cross the street without getting hit by a car, or solve a difficult math problem. But it turns out that minds aren't very good advisors when it comes to important but subjective matters. For example, minds are also responsible for some of the worst attributes of humanity: prejudice, hatred, stigma, suicide, homicide, and war, to name just a few. Thus, it's also important to understand that the mind has a personality of sorts, and these personality traits can make it difficult to handle in certain situations. In this section, we'll explore some of those personality traits and how they affect responses to stress.

The Mind Is a Control Freak

The mind believes that control is the answer for all of the big challenges you face in life: You need to control how you feel. You need to control what you think. You need to control memories you don't like. This is reflected in a phrase commonly used when someone is being too dramatic and emotional about something: "Control yourself, would you?" Control is in the water supply of our society. If you don't like having heartburn, there's a pill you can take to get rid of it. If you don't like having a headache, there's a pill for that too. And if you don't like being depressed or anxious, you can take a pill to get rid of those experiences. Our culture seems to have a pill for everything!

In fact, control is a hugely successful strategy for dealing with problems in the external world. The problem is, it's a total flop as a strategy for dealing with internal experiences like unpleasant emotions or stress reactions. For decades, it's been known that trying to control negative thoughts only makes those thoughts return with a vengeance (Wegner et al. 1987). Likewise, when you try to stifle or suppress emotions, those emotions just get more intense and seem out of control (Dunn et al. 2009). To add insult to injury, the emotion and thought control strategies that *do* work, such as alcohol, drugs, tobacco, bingeing, purging, and cutting, are almost always bad for you in the long run.

However, the mountain of information pointing to the futility of control won't deter your mind in the slightest. The mind will continue to tell you that the solution to your problems, including problems with stress, is to control how you feel and what you think, even if this means having to avoid or escape from situations that are producing these reactions. It will tell you that strong people can control their thoughts and feelings, and that you're weak if you can't. To the mind, the idea of just being an observer—just accepting the presence of emotions and thoughts—is nothing short of treason. We often joke with clients that the main problem with the mind is that it has a mind of its own!

The Mind Is Judgmental

When you're under stress, you might replay negative events over and over in your mind, such as situations where you feel you were treated unfairly or someone else was getting favored treatment and you weren't. The basic nature of the mind is to be judgmental. It categorizes, evaluates, compares, and predicts on a nonstop basis. It imposes its sense of moral order on the universe, and it becomes hyperactive when there's a violation of this order. An example would be receiving "undeserved" criticism from a teacher or supervisor. In situations like this, the mind will have you analyze why you're right and the other person is wrong, or why you're getting the short end of the stick compared to someone else.

The mind will also compare how you're doing in life compared to others or compared to how you think you should be doing. If you come up short in these comparisons, your mind will begin to analyze your flaws, why you have them, and how they're making you inferior to others. You can spend literally hours lost in what we call "analysis paralysis," ruminating about and replaying situations where you feel you've been mistreated. Because of its judgmental nature, the mind itself can become a continuous source of daily stress.

Mindfulness: The Antidote to the Mind

The uncomfortable truth is, we've become so reliant on our minds that we've forgotten that they aren't good for everything, including dealing with the problem of daily stress. In the previous chapter, we noted that one aspect of mindfulness is learning how to pay attention in a very specific way: nonjudgmentally, on purpose, and with a focus on the present moment. When you practice this type of mindful awareness, you'll immediately notice a number of qualitative shifts in how you relate to your mind.

The first and most important shift is realizing that although you have a mind, you are not the same as your mind. A good way to think about the relationship between you and your mind is that it's the speaker and you're the listener. Your mind speaks to you, and you hear what it says. You might even speak back to it! When you lose the distinction between you and your mind, which happens often when people are under stress, you start to respond to the mind's advice as if it's a command that you must follow. As a result, you might end up trying the same stress coping strategies over and over again, even though they aren't working.

The second major shift in how you relate to your mind is that, with mindfulness, you can recognize that the mind's messages can be either used or discarded, and that the choice is up to you. You are the human; the mind is the mind. A core feature of mindfulness is that you can see your mind's messages like information on a computer screen, weigh the merit of those messages, and then choose what to do, including following another path entirely. Your mind doesn't run the show; you do!

The final shift involves realizing that the mind doesn't know how to create vitality in life. The mind is indeed mindless in this way. We often remind clients that the mind doesn't do the present moment very well because it doesn't really have a role to play when people are just being here, now. It prefers to organize and execute daily habits automatically, without the need for participation from you, the human. So unless you consciously inject awareness into what you're doing in your daily routine, thereby creating a full mind, you lose contact with the vitality of the daily events and activities that make up the backbone of your existence. When people say something like "Just go out and smell the roses," they're really talking about turning off the mind's autopilot switch and adopting a deliberate, self-aware approach to daily life.

Restless Mind

Because your nervous system is driven by the dynamic balance between the fight-or-flight response of the SNS and the calming response of the PNS, you experience distinctly different states of mind depending upon which part of your nervous system is running the show. *Restless mind* is the term we use to describe the mental state when you're under stress and the SNS is activated. As the name implies, this mode of mind is characterized by hyperactivity, restlessness, low-grade anxiety, and a mild agitation that shows up whenever you stop moving and just stay still. The pace of mental activity in this state of mind is driven, and it's faster than most people like. People describe this experience in various ways, such as "I feel like I'm climbing the walls" or "I can't seem to get comfortable inside my skin."

Restless mind puts you in a self-protective stance where you're more prone to obsessing about what's wrong in your life. You're more likely to fixate on your past failings or worry about things in the future. You tend to see the negative side of any situation and magnify its impact, even if there are also positive aspects. Some of our clients have mentioned that it's almost like they're trying to find something to be negative about. Indeed, that's what this mode of mind has evolved to do. It's your brain's system for detecting and responding to threats to your survival and well-being. In a state of restless mind, it's hard to relax and sit still, even when the moment is right to do so.

Restless Mind's Advice: Control, Eliminate, or Avoid Stress

Restless mind evolved to detect and eliminate threats to your survival. Therefore, it takes a very predictable approach to solving the problem of stress and negative emotions, advising that you must eliminate the problem or control your emotional reactions to it to regain your health and well-being. This approach works well in the external world. For example, if you're out in a snowstorm and starting to get too cold, you need to get out of the storm and into a warm place. But it doesn't work well for solving problems in the inner world of emotional experience. For example, if you're feeling sad, it will advise that you need to do something that will make you happy so your sadness will go away. But unlike getting out of a snowstorm, you can't protect yourself from the causes of painful emotional states, such as losing a job, getting stuck in a traffic jam, or having someone break up with you.

Of course, the mind wants to succeed and therefore promotes a common but unfortunate behavior that makes it look like you're getting out of the snowstorm of emotions produced by stress. It's called *avoidance*, and restless mind specializes in this tactic. Avoidance means trying not to experience distressing internal events, such as sadness, painful memories, uncomfortable physical symptoms, or thoughts that provoke anger. With avoidance, you just don't think about these things, or if you do, you immediately distract yourself with something else. You might tell yourself that you aren't feeling sad when in fact you are feeling sad. You might drink alcohol or smoke pot to numb your awareness of what's going on inside. People have found a truly endless number of ways to avoid unpleasant emotions. The problem is, although avoidance creates the illusion that you're doing better, your stress-related problems will increase across the board. You can't solve any problem in your life while you're avoiding it.

Restless Mind Chatter

To compound the problems created by avoiding stress, restless mind offers seemingly nonstop advice and evaluations. One client remarked, "My mind never stops chattering at me. It's like it doesn't know how to shut up!" Indeed, you'll notice that restless mind is constantly commenting on how well you're doing a particular task, how pretty, thin, or well dressed you are compared to someone else, and on and on. Regardless of the topic, it never seems to tire of chattering, from the moment you wake up in the morning until you go to sleep at night.

Taking the mental chatter of restless mind seriously is definitely not good for you. For example, if you're feeling anxious about an upcoming work presentation, your mind will chatter at you about how important it is to not be anxious. When your anxiety persists, your mind will start to predict that you're going to have trouble because of your anxiety. When your anxiety gets even worse as a result, your mind will tell you that other people can control their anxiety, so why can't you? It will say this must mean there's something wrong with you and you need to figure out what it is or even worse things will happen to you. Over time, your attention will get completely sucked into your anxiety and your inability to control or eliminate it. The next strategy your mind will give you is a tactic to avoid having the anxiety, such as calling in sick or asking someone else to make the presentation.

The main problem with mental chatter is that the more you pay attention to it, the more chatter you get and the faster you get it. At a certain point, the mind's evaluations and directives start coming so fast that you can't think clearly, and tend to slip back into using the same strategies for avoiding stress over and over again.

Exercise: Identifying the Escape and Avoidance Strategies of Your Restless Mind

The urge to avoid or escape from something that's viewed as a threat to your welfare is hardwired into your nervous system. There's not a human being alive who isn't an escape artist, so to speak. While there are a seemingly unlimited number of escape tactics, our experience suggests that most people use a small number of preferred tactics repeatedly. We call these habitual responses "escape macros." These are well-practiced, automatic behaviors used to avoid making contact with painful stress reactions.

The purpose of this exercise is to introduce you to some of the more common escape macros and help you identify which you tend to use. We think it's useful to treat these habits in a lighthearted, even humorous way, rather than taking a heavy-handed, judgmental approach. If you can, just notice which of these escape macros applies to you. Although you can just let it go at that, we recommend that you write about any escape macros you use in your journal. For each, describe your specific strategies and what you're aware of while you're doing them. We'll help you deal with them later in this book.

The busy bee escapes from stress by staying busy all the time. If this is your main mode, most of the activities you engage in will be rather simple and require minimal awareness, like cleaning the countertops in the kitchen, mopping floors, or waxing the car. The busy bee moves quickly from one completed task to another and may sometimes repeat the same activity. The busy bee may also go overboard by making tasks larger than they need to be, for example, washing *all* of the towels in the entire house, even those that have barely been used. A more technical term for this escape routine is *activity defense*, with excess activity functioning to keep unpleasant stress reactions from seeping into awareness.

The butterfly shifts attention and focus constantly, like a butterfly flitting from bloom to bloom in a flower garden. This may occur with activities at work or at home. The butterfly starts activities, then quickly moves on to other activities, and then others. When sitting still, the butterfly often finds it difficult to focus on any one thing, making it difficult to do simple things such as reading a brief newspaper article or watching a TV program from beginning to end.

The ostrich ignores stress by not allowing any thoughts about it to creep into awareness. When others ask questions like "How are you doing?" the ostrich typically says, "Fine." Around others, the ostrich avoids participating in conversations that might trigger contact with stress responses that have been carefully buried. The ostrich often changes the subject if a partner or family member starts talking about stressors. The goal of the ostrich is to remain unaware of and out of contact with stress-related emotions.

The twiddler is a bundle of nervous energy. Unlike the busy bee, the twiddler doesn't engage in continuous activities and instead zones out in a rather limited space at home or at work. Whether seated, standing, or lying down, the twiddler's hands, arms, legs, or feet are usually in continuous motion. Anxious movements might include tapping a foot, twiddling fingers, mindlessly handling an object, hair twirling or pulling, or other small repetitive behaviors. The twiddler has a hard time staying in one position for very long and often alternates between sitting and standing. The twiddler uses these minor, repetitive behaviors to bleed off energy due to stress and keep stress-related emotions at bay.

The rationalizer is aware that stress is present but explains it away. The goal is to effectively disavow the existence of stress by insisting that it's something else—something much less serious. This is sometimes called denial, and it's a powerful defense against coming to grips with the reality that a problem is serious. The rationalizer may attempt to normalize the stressful situation (for example, thinking, *Anyone who's expected to work that many hours is bound to be pretty tired*); minimize the impact of the stress symptoms (*I can make it even if I'm only sleeping four hours a night; I just can double up on my energy drinks*); or compare the current stress level to that of others who "have it much worse." Usually, the rationalizer falls back on these strategies as a way to deflect the concern of others, such as a partner, friend, or coworker.

The busybody diverts attention away from personal stress by over-focusing on someone else, creating a lot of drama and emotional arousal around the other person's problems. Often this attention is directed at a family member with some type of substance abuse or behavioral problem. The busybody is often fixated on controlling the other person's behavior. This consumes most of the busybody's free time and mental energy, limiting opportunities for the busybody to directly experience stress.

The worrier escapes stress by worrying about anything and everything *other* than the stressful situation. Worrying all the time draws attention away from painful stress-related emotions. The worrier may not sleep well due to thinking about one worrisome topic after another into the wee hours of the night. Like the butterfly, the worrier tends to flit about, shifting from one worry to another when discussing concerns with a partner, friend, or coworker. Often, a stressful situation that's glaringly apparent to others is conspicuously absent in these conversations.

The stoic escapes stress-related emotions by bottling them up inside and often takes the stance that strong people don't show signs of stress. The stoic may even deny that stress is present. In fact, the stoic often denies having *any* emotional reactions and therefore may seem emotionally flat and numb. Topics that would typically give rise to emotions seem to have no impact on the stoic. Allowing even a trace of emotion to show up endangers the stoic's strategy of complete emotional shutdown.

The numbster will use any means necessary to numb out the effects of stress, from drinking excessively, using drugs, or overeating to gambling, cutting, or sleeping the day away. The guiding philosophy of the numbster's approach is that you can't feel something if you aren't there to feel it. This pattern of behavior often is accompanied by self-isolation.

***

As you review the results of this self-assessment, try to take a light-hearted approach. You aren't the only one out there who's practicing avoidance strategies, so the point isn't to compare yourself to others. Instead, we encourage you to remember the particular escape macros you tend to use. Then, when you notice that you're using them, silently say to yourself, "Right now, I'm being the stoic" (or whatever macro is appropriate). Being aware that you're avoiding a stressful emotion is often the first step in learning how to do something different.

Quiet Mind

As mentioned in the previous chapter, there's increasing reason to believe that using mindfulness techniques produces a distinctly different type of brain activity, characterized by unique electrical profiles. We like to call the experience of this alternative state of being *quiet mind*. In contrast to the pedal-to-the-metal experience of restless mind, it's characterized by a sense of being in the moment with no need to do anything other than be here now. Instead of anxiety, there's a sense of safety and self-acceptance. Instead of agitation, there's a sense of calmness and well-being.

The tradition of mindfulness is rich in anecdotal reports about the life-altering experience of being in contact with quiet mind. Generally, it involves developing a different kind of awareness, one that's completely present, expansive, calm, detached, and full of understanding. Lest you think this is the sole province of lifelong meditators, recall the study discussed in chapter 1, in which young college students with no prior mindfulness practice were able to induce this state of mind with only a brief regimen of mindfulness instruction.

The barriers to inducing a state of quiet mind aren't as formidable as you might think. Frankly, the biggest barrier you'll face is that you can get so busy interacting with restless mind that you don't have time left over to practice strategies that bring you into a state of quiet mind. This is why the lifestyle planning in part 3 of this book is so critical to transcending stress.

Once you understand that you don't have to be dominated and directed by restless mind, and that you don't have to escape or avoid the way you feel, you can devote yourself to building a mindfulness-based lifestyle. For example, you might make a conscious effort to develop daily routines that activate your PNS and produce a state of peace and self-acceptance.

There are many benefits to spending as much time as possible visiting quiet mind, largely due to the fact that unlike most of our daily experiences with the mind, quiet mind isn't really based in logic or rational thought. Quiet mind experiences tap into other forms of human knowing, such as intuition, inspiration, and transcendent awareness. Practicing this state of mind will help counterbalance restless mind's excessive emphasis on analysis, control, and judgment. In reality, there are many things we cannot know through rational analysis; we can only experience them directly in the moment, without any rational process to guide us.

Whereas restless mind wants to analyze and understand your problems in life, we want you to experience the sheer joy of being alive. In a state of quiet mind, you might experience an irrational but inherent sense of safety, joy, self-acceptance, well-being, and freedom. This is because PNS activation triggers the brain's reward centers, flooding the brain with naturally occurring opioids. When this part of your nervous system is activated, you're more likely to feel loved and whole inside, achieve some distance from unpleasant emotions, experience empathy and compassion for others (and yourself), and experience a sense of being connected to everyone and everything—not a bad place to be! These are the neural networks that have been targeted by meditative and mystical traditions through the centuries, and they're strengthened by brain training techniques you'll learn throughout the remainder of this book. So keep reading!

Gentle Reminders

In this chapter, we suggested that the mind is like the operating system of the brain. It functions in much the same way a computer operating system does, displaying messages on the computer screen of your awareness. We also suggested that the mind tends to have a distinct nature that isn't all that user-friendly. Under stress, the negative traits of mind tend to get exaggerated, resulting in restless mind, which is hyperactive, bossy, and judgmental. It views stress reactions and negative emotions as problems that must be solved by analysis, control, and willpower, even though these strategies fail miserably when it comes to dealing with stress-related emotions.

We also offered an antidote to restless mind: mindfulness, which can produce a state of quiet mind. Quiet mind will calm and settle your nervous system, and with a calm brain you can experience life directly. You'll also be able to adopt an open, accepting stance toward stressful events and take actions that are in alignment with what matters to you. Strategies for cultivating quiet mind are grossly underemphasized in our culture, particularly in comparison to the extensive training we receive encouraging us to live in the self-critical and self-rejecting grip of restless mind. Being human means learning to live with these two modes of mind and working with the dynamic tension that naturally exists between them.

In the next chapter, we'll introduce five specific qualities of living mindfully and help you assess your current capacity for each. You'll probably be pleased to find that you already have strengths in some of these areas. The information that you glean can help you zero in on the skills you need to develop. This will guide your practice when you get to part 2 of the book, in which we offer a wide variety of mindfulness techniques that will help you transcend daily stress and live a vital, purposeful life.

CHAPTER 3

The Five Facets of Mindfulness

The present moment is filled with joy and happiness.
If you are attentive, you will see it.

—Thich Nhat Hanh

The reality of daily stress is that, since you can't truly avoid it, you must learn to face it and use it to your advantage. This is like a mental version of the ancient martial art of jujitsu: you take the negative energy of stress and convert it into healthy, life-affirming experience. This practice of mental jujitsu involves being willing to disobey restless mind and its advice to escape from or avoid stress. When you follow this advice (and remember, you do get to choose), you end up headed down a path that encourages you to shut down emotionally and engage in all sorts of avoidance behaviors.

As an alternative, we want to help you develop your mental jujitsu skills so you can approach stressful situations, feel what you feel, and choose to take actions that promote your sense of well-being. Practicing mindfulness gives you another strategy to use when you're tempted to follow the ineffective rules of the restless mind.

In this chapter, we'll introduce you to five specific facets of mindfulness that will help you take a more quiet-mind approach to daily stress. We'll describe each facet of mindfulness in detail and provide some real-life examples of people with weaker and stronger skills in that area. This will give you a better sense of how each facet of mindfulness can positively impact the quality of your life. We'll also help you assess your skills in each skill area so you can determine your relative areas of strength and weakness. This will help you develop a more focused practice plan as you work your way through the rest of the book.

Mindfulness: A Diamond in the Rough

There has been an explosion of research into attention, mindfulness, and classical meditative practices in the last decade, and it is very exciting stuff indeed. Our particular approach is based on the work of Ruth Baer and colleagues at the University of Kentucky (Baer 2003; Baer et al. 2008). They administered several different surveys of attention and mindfulness to a large group of people and determined that there are five core aspects of an intentional, mindful approach to living. Our terms for these five facets are observing, describing, detaching, loving yourself, and acting mindfully. Studies of these five facets suggest that higher skill levels in these areas are associated with greater emotional intelligence, self-compassion, and openness to new learning opportunities.

In the self-assessments a bit later in this chapter, we use items from a survey developed by Baer and colleagues called the Five Facet Mindfulness Questionnaire (FFMQ; Baer et al. 2006). Like the individual facets of a beautiful diamond, each aspect of mindfulness makes a unique contribution to your ability to live mindfully. At the same time, just as no single facet defines the diamond's beauty, no single aspect of mindfulness practice is more important than another. When skills in each of these areas are operating in harmony with one another, the resulting improvements in your life will be much greater than what you'd experience by practicing any one technique alone. Finally, as with a diamond in the rough, you must hone and polish your skills through practice to really capitalize on the stress-reducing benefits of mindfulness. If you're interested in conducting follow-up self-assessments of your mindfulness skills over time, you can retake the assessments in this chapter periodically.

As mentioned, all of the following self-assessments use items from the Five Facet Mindfulness Questionnaire. We've provided a short version of the FFMQ in the appendix of this book, and two downloadable versions, the original and the short form, at http://www.newharbinger.com/31274 (see the back of this book for instructions on how to access them).

The goal of the self-assessments that follow (which are also available for download at http://www.newharbinger.com/31274) is to help you zero in on skills that you might want to improve with practice. If you're like most people, you may be somewhat reluctant to see the results of these assessments. Don't despair! You're likely to find that you already have some strong mindfulness skills in place. You just have to organize them into a tight, well-practiced routine so they become second nature in daily life.

Facet 1: Observe

Observing skills consist of being able to just notice things that are happening both inside you (physical sensations, thoughts, feelings, memories) and outside you (sounds, sights, colors, faces, others' activities). In observing mode, you hold still mentally and focus attention in a singular way, sort of like zooming in with camera lens.

People vary widely in their ability to observe different aspects of their internal or external world, and being an observer is easier in some situations than in others. For example, you may find it easy to tune in to bodily sensations but difficult to notice thoughts, feelings, or memories that show up in your mind's eye. Or you may be able to pay attention to sounds and colors in your environment but find it hard to direct your attention to internal sensations like breathing or your hands resting on the arm of a chair. Observing skills cover a lot of territory, inside and outside your body, and you may be able to use your strengths in one area to increase your abilities in other areas.

Exercise: Self-Assessment for Facet 1— Observe

Below is a collection of statements from the FFMQ that ask about your everyday experience in using observing skills. Using the scale of 1 to 5 below, indicate, on the line to the left of each statement, how frequently or infrequently you've had each experience in the last month.

Please answer according to what really reflects your experience rather than what you think your experience should be.

1 = *never or very rarely true*

2 = *not often true*

3 = *sometimes true, sometimes not true*

4 = *often true*

5 = *very often or always true*

_____ 1. When I'm walking, I deliberately notice the sensations of my body moving.

_____ 2. When I take a shower or a bath, I stay alert to the sensations of water on my body.

_____ 3. I notice how foods and drinks affect my thoughts, bodily sensations, and emotions.

_____ 4. I pay attention to sensations, such as the wind in my hair or sun on my face.

_____ 5. I pay attention to sounds, such as clocks ticking, birds chirping, or cars passing.

_____ 6. I notice the smells and aromas of things.

_____ 7. I notice visual elements in art or nature, such as colors, shapes, textures, or patterns of light and shadow.

_____ 8. I pay attention to how my emotions affect my thoughts and behaviors.

_____ Observe score

Take a moment to think about your strengths in this area. Do you find it easier to be an observer of your experience in some contexts than in others? Do you have some natural cues you use to help remind you to adopt the observer approach when you're stressed? People differ in these regards. Some people like to use a catchphrase, such as "Just notice, don't react," while others generate a mental image, like being a bird watcher looking at thoughts or emotions through binoculars, to help them kick into the observer mode.

After considering your strengths in this area, write a brief summary statement about those strengths in your journal. If you have ideas about particular situations where it's easier for you to activate your observing skills, note those as well.

Your responses to the eight statements above provide an estimate of your current ability to observe. The following two examples may also be helpful for giving you an idea of what different skill levels in observing look like in real life.

• Leslie: Limited Skills in Observing

Leslie found it very difficult to be aware of sensations within her body and had trouble being attentive to physical obstacles in her immediate environment. She often noticed cuts or bruises on her hands and arms but couldn't recall how or when they happened. Leslie's husband kidded her about being clumsy because she frequently bumped into household objects while lost in thought. When Leslie tried to tune in to herself, she often drew a blank. She couldn't identify any particular experiences inside her. To her, it seemed that most people were always talking about their feelings, and she envied them. Even when she tried, it was hard for her to be aware of any emotion except in situations that produced very strong reactions.

• Sam: Stronger Skills in Observing

Sam enjoyed observing from a young age. His relatives, particularly his grandfather, encouraged him to practice observing skills on a regular basis. As a five-year-old, he was able to spend ten or fifteen minutes watching an anthill and discussing his observations with his grandfather. His mother was an artist and encouraged him to stop and look at scenery as if he was going to paint a picture of it from memory. They often painted together, both landscapes and more abstract representations of emotions. Sam was quite introspective and spent a lot of time reflecting on how his daily life affected his emotions. He liked allowing his thoughts and memories to just come into his head while he watched.

Facet 2: Describe

Describing refers to your ability to use words to organize and convey what you're aware of either inside or outside you at any moment in time. Some people use the phrase "being a witness." The job of a witness is to tell the truth, the whole truth, and nothing but the truth. There are several core features of being a witness. First, witnessing must be anchored in the present moment as it unfolds in front of you. For example, witnessing involves being able to label a strong emotion, such as feeling intensely afraid as you begin to make a short public speech, in the moment you make contact with it.

Second, descriptions of direct experience should be as objective as possible. The witness doesn't interpret events but instead simply describes the event as fully as possible. Rather than making an evaluative statement about being afraid, the witness focuses on the immediate qualities present in the fear experience: "heart beating faster, breathing more shallow, thinking about not wanting to make a mistake." Finally, witnessing is an ongoing process, with new words being required as new experiences enter into your field of awareness, one after another.

Exercise: Self-Assessment for Facet 2 —Describe

Below is a collection of statements from the FFMQ that ask about your everyday experience in using describing skills. Using the scale of 1 to 5 below, indicate, on the line to the left of each statement, how frequently or infrequently you've had each experience in the last month.

Note that for questions 3, 4, and 5, you need to subtract the number associated with your answer from 6 to obtain the score for the item. For example, if your answer to statement 3 is 4 (often true), you'll subtract 4 from 6, resulting in a score of 2. Please answer according to what really reflects your experience rather than what you think your experience should be.

1 = never or very rarely true

2 = not often true

3 = sometimes true, sometimes not true

4 = often true

5 = very often or always true

____ 1. I'm good at finding words to describe my feelings.

____ 2. I can easily put my beliefs, opinions, and expectations into words.

6–____ ____ 3. It's hard for me to find the words to describe what I'm thinking.

6–____ ____ 4. I have trouble thinking of the right words to express how I feel about things.

6–____ ____ 5. When I have a sensation in my body, it's hard for me to describe it because I can't find the right words.

____ 6. Even when I'm feeling terribly upset, I can find a way to put it into words.

____ 7. My natural tendency is to put my experiences into words.

____ 8. I can usually describe how I feel at the moment in considerable detail.

____ Describe score

Take a moment to think about your strengths in this area. Do you find it easier to label your experience in some contexts than in others? Do some methods, such as writing, help you better label your experiences? People differ in these regards. Some people like to describe their experience to others, while others prefer to write their descriptions, and still others prefer to describe silently, without talking or writing.

After considering your strengths in this area, write a brief summary statement about those strengths in your journal. If you have ideas about particular situations where it's easier for you to activate your describing skills, note those as well.

Your responses to the eight statements above provide an estimate of your current ability to describe. The following two examples may also be helpful for giving you an idea of what different skill levels in describing look like in real life.

• Steve: Limited Skills in Describing

Steve found it difficult to put his thoughts into words. In school, he'd struggled with any subject that required him to observe and describe things in the outer world, from art class to biology. When asked what he was thinking about, Steve typically answered, "I don't know. Nothing, I guess." Even when he tried to write his thoughts, as a friend suggested, he usually drew a blank. He also struggled with being able to label his emotions, particularly feelings of fear and sadness. When he felt those emotions, he tended to become tongue-tied. So instead of looking at them or thinking about them, he tried to ignore them or to use alcohol to numb his awareness of what was going on inside. So many things seemed to set off Steve's emotions, and he believed he must be different from most people, who seemed to be generally calm and happy. He was taking a variety of prescribed antidepressant medications, but he kept turning to alcohol more than he cared to in an effort to keep his feelings at bay.

• Regan: Stronger Skills in Describing

Regan, a young married woman with children, enjoyed gardening and art. She seemed to thrive in situations that required social contact and getting to know others. Even when she was sad about something, she liked to express these feelings to others, and sharing with others in this way usually gave her more clarity about her emotions. She felt things deeply, and she'd always found it helpful to talk about her feelings with a close friend or relative. When she was troubled by something, she usually sought out a trusted friend for a long conversation about her thoughts and feelings. In these conversations, she preferred to just talk and have her friend just listen. Given how important this was to her psychological well-being, Regan cultivated relationships that could support this type of interaction.

Facet 3: Detach

For the facet of describing, we distinguished between descriptive words that are closely tied to direct qualities of experience and evaluative words that assign positive or negative meaning to experiences. While we encourage you to develop and use your describing abilities, no amount of practice will silence restless mind's insistence on displaying powerful and provocative messages on your mind's computer screen. The antidote is to practice detachment. Detachment functions much like the Teflon coating on a frying pan, allowing food particles that would otherwise stick to the pan to slide right off. With detachment, instead of letting restless mind's evaluations, predictions, and comparisons stick to you, you just let them slide off.

Detaching means allowing thoughts, feelings, memories, and sensations to simply be present without becoming hooked by mental evaluations of what you're aware of, such as *I shouldn't be feeling sad; look at everything I've got to be happy about.* Another term people often use to describe the act of detaching is "letting go." When you let go, you ignore the temptation to hold on to something that causes you to suffer. This is difficult to do, particularly when thoughts are compelling, feelings are painful, or memories make you feel like you're reliving the past. Most of us want to avoid pain and suffering and have escape strategies for doing just that. Detachment skills help us develop the ability to stay present with unpleasant internal experiences without getting hooked by them.

Exercise: Self-Assessment for Facet 3— Detach

Below is a collection of statements from the FFMQ that ask about your everyday experience in using detaching skills. Using the scale of 1 to 5 below, indicate, on the line to the left of each statement, how frequently or infrequently you've had each experience in the last month. Please answer according to what really reflects your experience rather than what you think your experience should be.

1 = never or very rarely true

2 = not often true

3 = sometimes true, sometimes not true

4 = often true

5 = very often or always true

_____ 1. I perceive my feelings and emotions without having to react to them.

_____ 2. I watch my feelings without getting lost in them.

_____ 3. In difficult situations, I can pause without immediately reacting.

_____ 4. When I have distressing thoughts or images, I am able just to notice them without reacting.

_____ 5. When I have distressing thoughts or images, I feel calm soon after.

_____ 6. _When I have a distressing thought or image, I sit back and am aware of the thought or image without getting taken over by it._

_____ 7. _When I have distressing thoughts or images, I just notice them and let them go._

_____ _Detach score_

Take a moment to think about your strengths in this area. Do you find it easier to detach in some contexts than in others? For example, is it easier to detach when a coworker makes a snide remark than it is when your spouse criticizes your appearance? Are there mental cues you use to remind yourself to detach when you're getting hooked by your reactions to a stressful situation or interaction, such as "Just let go"?

After considering your strengths in this area, write a brief summary statement about those strengths in your journal. If you have ideas about particular strategies or situations that make it easier for you to activate your detachment skills, note those as well.

Your responses to the seven statements above provide an estimate of your current ability to detach. The following two examples may also be helpful for giving you an idea of what different skill levels in detaching look like in real life.

• Ben: Limited Skills in Detaching

Ben was a single father with one child, his son Charlie. Ben and Charlie had always liked the same things when Charlie was younger. But as Charlie grew into adolescence, he pulled away from Ben and started to hang out with a rough crowd. Eventually, Charlie was arrested for possession of drugs, which broke Ben's heart.

Afterward, Ben began to experience problems in numerous areas of his life. He couldn't concentrate on his work because of his guilt feelings. Often, he'd lie awake at night thinking back on what might have gone wrong. He tried to figure out how he had failed Charlie to the extent that Charlie had turned to drugs. He became preoccupied with Charlie's problems and kept bringing the topic up with friends, who urged Ben to remind himself that he'd done the best he could as a father. Eventually, he fell so far behind on work projects that he lost some contracting jobs. He went to his doctor looking for help, complaining, "I can't get my mind to turn off."

• Lilly: Stronger Skills in Detaching

Lilly was a new mother. She had dreamed of being a mother ever since she received her first doll as a small child. After her baby was born, she noticed that she was getting wound up about having everything in its place, keeping her home free of germs, and being on guard for things that might pose a risk to her daughter's safety. To compensate, she decided to spend ten to fifteen minutes every morning thinking about her daughter with no particular goal in mind. During these times, she encouraged herself to notice her thoughts with a sense of curiosity and to let go of any judgments her mind offered about her abilities as a young mother.

She had used a similar technique in college, when she struggled with perfectionism and felt so discouraged about her ability to excel in school that she sought help for depression. Now, even though Lilly sometimes experienced anxiety and fear related to images of her daughter sustaining some type of injury due to her neglect or lack of foresight, she was able to help her mind find some peace when these images presented themselves. Over time, she started to notice that she was better able to handle other types of stress-producing thoughts and reactions in her daily life. It seemed that learning to detach from anxiety-provoking images about her daughter transferred to other emotionally charged situations in her daily life.

Facet 4: Love Yourself

The ability to show love and kindness to yourself is a powerful tool for creating a state of quiet mind. It's an important concept in Buddhist writings about human suffering and the path out of that suffering. Loving yourself, which is sometimes referred to as *self-compassion*, is garnering increasing attention in psychological theories of health, well-being, and spirituality. Self-compassion isn't self-centeredness, self-pity, or self-indulgence. In fact, self-compassion makes it easier to extend love and compassion to others. It's an unconditional attitude of deep respect that doesn't depend on your performance or accomplishments and doesn't rely on approval from others. It means showing concern for your own well-being, being sensitive to your own distress, tolerating that distress without self-criticism or judgment, seeking to understand the causes of your distress, and doing all of this with a sense of warmth and gentleness.

While the typical social training encourages us to practice kindness toward others, we tend to be leery about being too kind and forgiving toward ourselves. We've been socialized to believe that constant self-criticism is necessary if we are to succeed and move up the pecking order. In addition, we tend to believe we need to prove our worth by being better than others and refusing to accept personal failures. These are just some of the reasons why there's hardly a more damning criticism than to be called selfish. Being products of this same cultural tradition, we the authors actually debated using the label "love yourself" because we worried it might trigger an automatic response of "What! That's selfish of me and dangerous for others!" If this rings true for you, please experience it with detachment and read on.

Exercise: Self-Assessment for Facet 4— Love Yourself

Below is a collection of statements from the FFMQ that ask about your everyday experiences with loving yourself. Using the scale of 1 to 5 below, indicate, on the line to the left of each statement, how frequently or infrequently you've had each experience in the last month. Note that for all of the items you need to subtract the number associated with your answer from 6 to obtain the score. For example, if your answer to statement 1 is 2 (not often true), you'll subtract 2 from 6, resulting in a score of 4. Please answer according to what really reflects your experience rather than what you think your experience should be.

1 = *never or very rarely true*

2 = *not often true*

3 = *sometimes true, sometimes not true*

4 = *often true*

5 = *very often or always true*

6–____ ____ 1. I criticize myself for having irrational or inappropriate emotions.

6–____ ____ 2. I tell myself that I shouldn't be feeling the way I'm feeling.

6–____ ____ 3. I believe that some of my thoughts are abnormal or bad and I shouldn't think that way.

6–____ ____ 4. I make judgments about whether my thoughts are good or bad.

6–____ ____ 5. I tell myself I shouldn't be thinking the way I'm thinking.

6–____ ____ 6. I think some of my emotions are bad or inappropriate and I shouldn't feel them.

6–____ ____ 7. I disapprove of myself when I have irrational ideas.

6–____ ____ 8. When I have distressing thoughts or images, I judge myself as good or bad, depending on what the thought or image is about.

____ Loving yourself score

Take a moment to think about your strengths in this area. Do you find it easier to show kindness to yourself in some situations and more difficult in others? For example, is it easier to care for yourself when you've worked hard and feel physically exhausted, and more difficult when you've missed a deadline because you simply forgot about it? Do you have any mental or verbal cues that remind you to take it easy on yourself when you aren't doing well, such as "No one is perfect"?

After considering your strengths in this area, write a brief summary statement about those strengths in your journal. If there have been times in your life when you were less critical and more accepting of yourself, write about that in your journal as well, as it may provide some clues about how to reactivate that ability.

Your responses to the eight statements above will give you an estimate of your current ability to love yourself. The following two examples may also be helpful for giving you an idea of what different levels of skill with this facet look in like in real life.

• Betty: Limited Skills in Self-Compassion

Betty grew up with critical parents. They believed that constantly pointing out her shortcomings would help her build character and determination. She incorporated these beliefs into her way of motivating herself and took pride in her accomplishments. She went to college on an athletic scholarship and was the first in her family to graduate from college. Her internal critic played a role in her success, but it came at a price. As the demands of her athletic and academic activities grew, her self-criticism and refusal to accept anything less than perfection from herself also grew.

Her internal critic started to focus on her weight and physical appearance, even though she was in great shape physically, and eventually she couldn't stand to look at herself in a mirror. She always focused on the parts of her body that she didn't like. She eventually developed eating problems, alternating between periods of restricting her eating and losing weight and periods of binge eating and weight gain. Whether she was losing or gaining, Betty couldn't accept herself, and in time she lost confidence even in areas where she excelled. She compared herself to other women in terms of looks, body shape, intelligence, and happiness, and always found herself wanting. Ultimately, she developed problems with depression.

• Jerry: Stronger Skills in Self-Compassion

Even as a young boy, Jerry seemed to be able to make lemons into lemonade. When he broke his leg on the first day of football season in high school, he decided to become the unofficial mascot of his team. When his high school sweetheart broke up with him after graduation, he was devastated, but he decided to proceed with his plan to enroll in a vocational training program and eventually became a diesel mechanic.

Jerry started smoking when he was fourteen. His best friend, Les, sneaked a pack of his parents' cigarettes out of the house, and they smoked a few together in the woods behind Les's house. Jerry felt really sick, but somehow he liked it enough to try it again. He became a pack-a-day smoker and kept up that habit for twenty years. His doctors repeatedly told him to quit, and he knew he should because it was impairing his fitness, which was important to him for pursuing outdoor activities like hunting, fishing, and camping. He tried to quit a number of times, and one time he was successful for over four months before he started smoking again.

The next time Jerry tried to stop smoking, he decided to use an Internet program to support his effort, and it helped him gain some insight about a pattern he'd fallen into around quitting: criticizing himself for even having an urge to smoke. When he felt those urges, he tended to tell himself things like *You'll never make it*, *You've got to smoke or you'll go crazy*, or *What's wrong with you?* So he decided to take the same approach to quitting smoking as he did with the rest of his life, which he summed up with this motto: Do the best you can and let the cards fall where they may. He noticed that this approach allowed him to make room for urges to smoke and to just do the best he could in those moments. With that approach, he finally succeeded in quitting.

Facet 5: Act Mindfully

Acting mindfully means being aware of what you're doing as you're doing it. This is sometimes called "acting with intention." It means being squarely located the present moment and behaving in a way that reflects your beliefs and principles. This is a very different way of living than the autopilot approach we described earlier, where you perform daily routines without a real sense of engagement.

But even if you turn off the autopilot switch, there's no guarantee you'll choose to act with intention. You might still act impulsively in many ways: eating too much, drinking too much, talking too much, spending too much, staying up too late, and on and on. Acting mindfully is especially difficult when you're besieged by stress reactions such as negative thoughts, painful feelings, unpleasant memories, or distressing physical symptoms. At these times, you're most prone to engaging in impulsive behaviors to avoid mental reactions to stress; for example, you might drink too much to quiet anxiety symptoms.

Exercise: Self-Assessment for Facet 5— Act Mindfully

Below is a collection of statements from the FFMQ that ask about your everyday experience with acting mindfully. Using the scale of 1 to 5 below, indicate, on the line to the left of each statement, how frequently or infrequently you've had each experience in the last month. Note that for all of the items you need to subtract the number associated with your answer from 6 to obtain the score. For example, if your answer to statement 1 is 2 (not often true), you'll subtract 2 from 6, resulting in a score of 4. Please answer according to what really reflects your experience rather than what you think your experience should be.

1 = never or very rarely true

2 = not often true

3 = sometimes true, sometimes not true

4 = often true

5 = very often or always true

6-____ ____ 1. I find it difficult to stay focused on what's happening in the present.

6-____ ____ 2. It seems I am "running on automatic" without much awareness of what I'm doing.

6-____ ____ 3. I rush through activities without being really attentive to them.

6-____ ____ 4. I do jobs or tasks automatically, without being aware of what I'm doing.

6-____ ____ 5. I find myself doing things without paying attention.

6-____ ____ 6. When I do things, my mind wanders off and I'm easily distracted.

6-____ ____ 7. I don't pay attention to what I'm doing because I'm daydreaming, worrying, or otherwise distracted.

6-____ ____ 8. I am easily distracted.

____ Act mindfully score

Take a moment to think about your strengths in this area. Do you find it easier to act mindfully in some situations and more difficult in others? For example, is it easier for you to show up for a talk with your spouse when you take a walk together? Is it more difficult for you to maintain your attention on a task when you're worried about a personal problem? Do you have any strategies that help you focus your attention or that help you experience impulses without acting on them?

After considering your strengths in this area, write a brief summary statement about those strengths in your journal. If you have ideas about particular situations where it's easier for you to employ your skills in acting mindfully, note those as well.

Your responses to the eight statements above provide an estimate of your current ability to act mindfully. The following two examples may also be helpful for giving you an idea of what different skill levels in acting mindfully look like in real life.

• Annie: Limited Skills in Acting Mindfully

Annie worked as an administrative assistant in a small office. She'd held her job for over ten years and for the most part had met her performance evaluation goals every year, even though her supervisor always indicated a need for improvement in several areas. Usually, the areas of concern involved Annie seeming distracted and not picking up on anything new or outside her routine.

Annie felt like she was going through the motions often when she was at work, particularly over the past year, after her husband left for an extended military deployment. She eventually received a warning from her supervisor that she would be let go if she kept making errors in her reports. Annie wanted to keep her job, especially because her family needed the money, but she just didn't know how to become more focused at work. At home, life seemed like a blur. She raced from task to task and rarely took time to just be with her two teenage sons. She often ate in the kitchen while doing the dishes or cooking meals for her sons.

• Victor: Stronger Skills in Acting Mindfully

Victor struggled to finish high school because he got caught up in a group of rowdies and didn't attend class regularly or finish homework assignments. He married while in college, started a family, and just barely managed to earn his degree. After graduating, he quickly got a job working as a laborer on a residential construction crew. While he made decent money and was able to support his wife and two children, he didn't feel at all challenged by the work. He had always dreamed of being an information technology specialist. Even during his high school days, he was fascinated by computers, software, and networks.

Eventually, Victor made the decision to begin saving money from each paycheck to fund a switch to a new career. He checked out a few vocational training programs and, after consulting with his wife, applied to one and was accepted. He took a night job to cover family expenses and went to school during the day. He enjoyed every minute of his training; he did extracurricular reading of technical manuals and often stayed after class to pick the brains of his instructors.

After getting his degree, Victor found it difficult to break into the IT community. The economy was poor and jobs were scarce, but he kept refreshing his résumé and considered every type of employment in his new field, including part-time work. He kept reminding himself that he had gifts in computer science and would eventually find a way to share it with people who would benefit from his skills. He eventually got a part-time IT job at a local health care center. The day he was hired was the most rewarding day of his life, and he took his wife out to dinner to celebrate the beginning of his new career.

Exercise: Creating Your Mindfulness Profile and Setting Targets for Practice

Before reading on, take a moment to summarize your assessment results. This will create a profile of your mindfulness skills. Record your scores for each facet below. Notice that we provide space for your scores in three months. At that time, we'd like you to take these self-assessments again to help gauge your progress with the brain training approach we outline in part 2 of the book. While it's reasonable to expect to make progress in three months, you may see improvements much sooner.

Mindfulness Profile Summary

Observe	Score today: _____	Score in three months: _____
Describe	Score today: _____	Score in three months: _____
Detach	Score today: _____	Score in three months: _____
Love yourself	Score today: _____	Score in three months: _____
Act mindfully	Score today: _____	Score in three months: _____

Take some time to reflect on your scores and, for each, imagine what it would look like if your skills were stronger than they are today. For example, let's say that you have a decent score for the observing facet of mindfulness. What would it be like to have a super high score, where you could practice observing even in the most stress-producing situations? Maybe you registered a lower score on the facet of loving yourself. Can you imagine what it would be like if you were much better at forgiving yourself or giving yourself credit when you need to? It never hurts to imagine a future in which you're even better at a skill than you are now.

Now we'd like you to develop a plan for increasing your skills in one or more of the facets of mindfulness covered in the assessments in this chapter. The chapters in part 2 of the book are organized in the same order as the assessments you just completed. If you have limited time to devote to brain training, for now you might plan to target one or two of the chapters in part 2 that you feel will be most helpful for you. You can start by reading the chapters that align with your targets, or just go through all of the chapters in sequence. Either way, in the long run it's best to read through all of the chapters and practice all of the exercises. Even if you have strong skills in one area, it can't hurt to make them even stronger! But for now, choose one or two areas you'll target as you begin your journey toward transcending stress.

My mindfulness practice areas are _____ and
_____ .

Tracking and Maintaining Your Mindfulness Skills Over the Long Haul

As mentioned, we've provided a short version of the Five Facet Mindfulness Questionnaire in the appendix, and two downloadable versions, the original and the short form, at http://www.newharbinger .com/31274. We recommend that you complete the short version during the first week of January every year as part of your New Year's resolutions. Doing so will help you quickly check in on the stability of your gains in mindfulness. If you notice that you're slipping in one or more areas, you might want to return to the corresponding chapter in part 2 of the book and redouble your efforts in practicing its exercises.

Also, bear in mind that having the support of others can be immensely helpful in sticking with your practice. When you make a commitment and share it with others, you'll probably feel more accountable. If you like, you can even ask others to support you in your practice by asking you for an update on a regular basis.

Gentle Reminders

In this chapter, we introduced you to the five facets of mindfulness: observe, describe, detach, love yourself, and act mindfully. Each contributes in a different way to developing a mindfulness-based lifestyle that will help you transcend daily stress. Thus, it's important to improve your strength in all five areas through daily practice. Remember, practice doesn't make perfect, but it does make permanent, strengthening skills and making them less likely to fade over time. We also asked you to complete a series of assessments of your skills in these areas. In all likelihood, the results of your self-assessments were uneven. This is fine; most people are stronger in some areas than in others. Use your results to help you target one or two facets of mindfulness to focus on as you work through part 2 of the book.

In part 2, our goal is to investigate each facet of mindfulness in more depth, both from a neuroscience perspective and in terms of personal impacts. We'll provide a host of brain training exercises and mindfulness practices that you can use to hone and polish your mindfulness skills until each facet shines beautifully in your life!

PART 2

Five Steps to Transcending Stress

CHAPTER 4

Observe

The faculty of voluntarily bringing back a wandering attention, over and over again, is the very root of judgment, character, and will.

—William James

In part 1 of the book, we described mindfulness as learning to pay attention on purpose and in a particular way. In this chapter, you'll start learning, in depth, about this special way of paying attention and how to use it in your daily life. The ability to focus your attention—the observe facet of the mindfulness diamond—is a fundamental skill for transcending daily stress, and you need to practice it regularly. When you practice observing, you activate brain circuits responsible for centering you mentally and focusing your attention. This ability to stay centered and focused allows you to respond more effectively to your own emotions and to the stresses you face (Tang et al. 2007).

Learning to focus your attention is important because when you're under stress, your attention tends to splinter. You may find that you lose your focus and jump from one thing to another as the physical arousal of stress activates restless mind. As a result, you'll tend to experience low-grade anxiety that can be quite unpleasant, especially when you're trying to relax, enjoy yourself, or even just get a good night's sleep. This overactivation of your nervous system and the persistent shifts of attention it creates can make you less organized and effective in responding to daily stress. Thus, learning to dial in your attention to what's happening within you or in the outside world is a key skill for mastering stress. This is a difficult task, particularly when you're stressed, but as you strengthen your observer skills, you'll be increasingly able to face stress without overreacting to it. This will help you activate quiet mind and choose more effective actions.

Core Observer Skills

Two aspects of being an observer are especially important, and we'll focus on both in this chapter. One quality is *centering*, in which you pull yourself out of distraction and reorganize your attention. Centering can involve an act as simple as closing your eyes, taking a few deep breaths, clearing your mind of clutter, and then opening your eyes again with newfound focus. Think of it this way: because attention is a limited resource, you first have to bring it back together in your mind. It only takes seconds to center yourself, but it won't happen automatically unless you practice doing it.

The second aspect of being an observer is *focusing*—applying your attention in a focused way on just one thing. Focused attention is like a laser beam that you point with extreme accuracy on a target. In addition to directing your attention accurately, it also involves keeping your attention on the target for as long as you want. When these two aspects of observing—centering and focusing—combine in the moment, you can (figuratively speaking) stare a hole in the stress-producing situation in front of you.

From Participant to Observer

Being an observer requires that you orient toward something that catches your interest, approach it, and pay attention to it. Just for fun, try that now. Find something in your immediate environment that interests you, then keep your attention focused on it for a minute or so. Notice what happens. Do you have the urge to look at something else? Does your mind distract you into thinking about something else? If you notice your attention shifting, can you redirect it back to the object of interest? In a nutshell, these are the skills it takes to be an observer.

Our minds are capable of taking three different perspectives on our immediate experience: participant, participant-observer, and observer. We spend almost all of our waking hours shifting between these three perspectives. None of them is better than the others; the key is learning how to shift between perspectives intentionally so you can use the perspective that works best in each situation. To help you get a better feel for how different these perspectives are, let's apply them to the experience of a roller coaster at an amusement park.

If you take the participant perspective, you climb into the front car of the roller coaster and take the ride with the sole intent of thrill seeking. You directly experience the excitement and terror of the ride. You aren't interested in anyone else who's riding with you; it's all about your immediate experience. In the participant perspective, the more you get into the ride, the better.

If you take the participant-observer perspective, you also hop on the roller coaster, but this time you're both experiencing the thrills and paying attention to the reactions of your fellow riders. Your attention is divided between your direct experience of being on the roller coaster and noticing all of the different verbal and nonverbal reactions of your fellow riders. Your reactions might even be influenced by what you see your fellow riders doing, for example, throwing your arms in the air and screaming as you plunge downward.

If you take the observer perspective, you don't actually get on the roller coaster. Rather, you position yourself so you can see all aspects of the roller coaster in a bigger context, such as how the platform and rails are designed, how the ride is powered, how people position themselves in the cars, and the various emotional reactions visible on the faces of the riders. The goal of the observer is to take in and process the entire context of the experience. This perspective allows you to see what's coming long before the riders, including how the ride will eventually end.

As you can see, simply observing a roller coaster is completely different than the experience of taking a ride on a roller coaster. Similarly, the experience of being a participant in a stressful situation is somewhat different than being a participant-observer, where you observe both yourself and others as you participate in a situation. And it's extremely different from the observer stance, where you focus exclusively on observing your internal and external experience without reacting to it.

As mentioned previously, there's no right way to experience life events; sometimes you'll want to be in participant mode, like when you're going to an amusement park just to have fun. The key is to be able to shift between perspectives when you need to. For example, stress tends to draw you into participant mode, so you end up absorbed in your emotions, thoughts, and physical reactions. When stress shows up, it's best to immediately shift into observer mode so you can avoid acting in ways that make your stress worse, such as ruminating about a stressful interaction or getting hooked by your anger over a real or perceived slight. In this chapter, we'll teach you skills that will help you intentionally adopt the observer stance, an approach that's essential to healthy functioning in response to daily stress.

The Neuroscience of Observing

Stress tends to trigger a very narrow form of awareness called *bottom-up attention*. Bottom-up attention originates in the core structures of the limbic system and evolved to help us scan for immediate threats to our survival. In this mode, you tend to focus attention on negative information and either ignore or disregard positive information. This is the default mode of attention produced by stress unless you consciously shift out of it. This is why people complain that stress interferes with their ability to think and make decisions. In essence, they're forced to use a lower form of attention to perform tasks that require higher-order attention. This mismatch contributes to the likelihood of making errors of judgment or reacting impulsively to stressful situations.

Fortunately, there's a counterbalancing type of attention that allows you to remain flexible and effective even when stressed. This mode, called *top-down attention*, originates in the insula, a higher-order brain structure. Top-down attention allows you to shift your attention inward so you can monitor and regulate how your body is reacting to stress, tuning in to your heart rate, respiration rate, muscle tension, and so on. With this type of attention your senses are more acute, so you might be aware of sounds or sights you wouldn't notice with bottom-up attention. Shifting to top-down attention is the first step in the process of regulating negative emotions produced by stress. You have to be aware of how you're feeling before you can do something about how you're feeling. Another benefit of top-down attention is that it allows you to visualize solutions to stress-producing problems and to maintain your focus on implementing those solutions even in the face of distractions.

The Neuroscience of Observing

The core skills involved in observing, the underlying neural circuits, and the associated mental processes are outlined below. It's important to understand that multiple sites in the higher-order regions of the brain interact in unison to produce a mental phenomenon like top-down attention. That's why this form of attention is also much more dynamic and flexible in addressing life situations that produce stress.

Observing skill: Centering

Areas of the brain involved

- Cortical midline structures, including the

- Anterior and posterior cingulate cortex, and the

- Dorsomedial and medial prefrontal cortex

Mental processes

- Orienting and organizing attention resources via breath control

- Generating self-referential verbal cues to focus

Observing skill: Focusing

Areas of the brain involved

- Intraparietal cortex

- Superior frontal cortex

- Insula

Mental processes

- Maintaining the focus of attention on a single mental event or object

- Shifting between inward-focused and outward-focused attention

Brain Training

When you learned to ride a bicycle, you probably learned it one step at a time. This is the way we'll teach you to become a better observer. In many ways, the steps are remarkably similar: You began with the intention to ride a bicycle, found a bike, and started by sitting on it with the kickstand down. You may have had to adjust the seat to find the right height for you. Then you learned to roll forward and operate the pedals and brakes, thereby adjusting your speed. All the while, you were learning how to balance yourself because without balance, you can't ride a bike. For better and worse, falling is an essential part of learning how to achieve balance.

Like learning to ride a bike, acquiring observer skills begins with establishing a regular practice time in a setting that promotes focusing, preferably a quiet location free from distractions. All of the following exercises will help you develop the ability to activate your innate top-down attention skills. Later, you can add other observer skills, such as shifting focus from one object of attention to another. Eventually, you'll notice that you're able to deploy observer skills with little conscious effort, a state a being centered and focused referred to as *effortless attention*. This will you help you access quiet mind when daily stresses start to add up.

Practice: Clearing Breath

As mentioned previously, centering is the first thing you need to do to enter into observer mode. Perhaps you've seen a concert pianist getting centered at the keyboard before starting a piece, or world-class athletes center themselves just prior to performing an athletic feat. What do you remember seeing them do? Typically, it involves taking a few deep breaths, often with your eyes disengaged and looking down. We call this the clearing breath, and it's something you can practice at any time during your day. It honestly takes just thirty seconds to clear your mind of distractions and center yourself by taking a few long, deep breaths.

To practice centering breath, slowly inhale for four to five seconds, pause for one second, and then slowly exhale slowly for four to five seconds. When you inhale, you might want to say something under your breath like "Relax"; then when you exhale, you might say something to yourself like "Focus." Repeat this sequence three times, then look up and see what a difference a few breaths can make!

Practice: Attending to Your Senses

This simple five- to ten-minute exercise is a good way to develop more skill in focusing your attention inward. It involves observing most of the basic senses that make up human perceptual experience: sight, sound, touch, and smell. These sensations are occurring all the time either inside or outside your body.

To practice, you can do this exercise with your eyes either open or closed, or with a combination of eyes open and closed, depending on what helps you focus best. To do this exercise, simply work through each sense as outlined below, taking about two minutes to practice observing each.

Vision. Start by just letting yourself notice anything that draws your interest. Once you lock in on something, try to see it with increasingly focused attention. This isn't a stare down in which your eyes water because you're staring without blinking. Rather, simply fix your attention on a single thing and take in the richness of color, hue, contrast, and other visual aspects of the object. We sometimes call this inhaling what you're aware of. Inhale it and roll it around in your mind's eye. Try to notice something about the object that you hadn't noticed before. You might even look at your hand or some other part of your body and just notice it.

Hearing. This is usually best done with eyes closed, as sight tends to override hearing. Try to listen for sounds inside your body, perhaps your heart beating or the sound of your breath moving in and out. Again, inhale what you're hearing and keep it in your mind's eye. Don't jump to something else you hear; just stay focused on whatever sound inside of you that you lock onto. After a while, turn your hearing outward and see if you pick up on a sound you hadn't noticed before. You may automatically hear something that's louder than other sounds. We encourage you to drop that sound and find another one that's less obvious. Keep your attention focused on that sound and notice what it sounds like when you're fully engaged.

Touch. Touch is such an interesting perception because it allows you to gauge temperature, pressure, and texture. Air is actually touching your nostrils as you breath in through your nose. You can notice the temperature of the air as it enters and the differing temperature as it exits. Another example is physical sensations like the feeling of your chest moving out and in as you breathe. You can also focus on external touch sensations, like the weight of your hands or the textures they feel. You can even experience the sensation of your entire body interfacing with the surface you're lying or sitting on. Try shifting your attention among various sectors of your body and just notice the sensations created as you change body positions.

Smell. Smells are all around us, but we seldom pay attention to them. With eyes closed, see if you can pick up a very faint smell in your environment. This can require some patience because we're conditioned to detect strong smells and let subtler ones pass. However, we are capable of latching onto subtle smells as well. Sometimes this works better initially if you create an opportunity to encounter aromas, perhaps smelling a flower or a fruit with a fairly faint aroma.

You may wonder about the fifth sense: taste. The nice thing about taste is that you get to use this sense in very focused moments during a typical day, each time you eat or drink. Thus, each time you begin to consume food or a beverage, you have an opportunity to work your taste buds. See if you can slow down the process of eating or drinking enough that you can savor specific tastes as they show up in your awareness. Eating a peach can be life-altering if you allow your attention to closely follow the flavors and your experience from beginning to end. Imagine the treat in store for you if you approach each bite of food with the goal of separating out distinct taste sensations. Try to describe these experiences out loud as you have them, as though you were a professional taste tester, hired to detect each nuance of flavor.

Practice: Shifting from Outward to Inward Focusing

Learning to flexibly shift attention from external to internal is another basic observer skill. One way to build this skill is to practice shifting your focus from an object in your environment, such as a chair or painting, to an internal stimulus, such as the sensation of breathing or the experience of having a tongue. You can choose anything to focus on, externally or internally, and you can vary what you focus on from day to day. You simply need to set an intention regarding specific external and internal things to focus on for your practice period and then stay with that intention.

To practice you'll need an external prompt, such as a timer or phone alarm, to initiate each shift. Set the timer for one to two minutes, then simply shift your attention back and forth, from internal to external, whenever the alarm goes off. This exercise will help you develop the ability to let go of one object of focus and approach another with flexibility and intention, so it's optimal to practice several such attention shifts during a practice period.

Practice: Observing Emotional Experiences

Emotions play a major role in motivating behavior. Sometimes they may stimulate prosocial behavior, and sometimes they may exacerbate the pain and frustration of daily hassles. Learning to observe your emotions with interest and curiosity will give you new tools for responding to stress creatively. People vary widely in their ability to notice and accept emotions, so be patient with yourself if this practice is difficult for you.

To practice, simply sit quietly and notice each emotion as it shows up in awareness. You might even think of an emotional event in your life to bring up emotions. When you notice an emotion, explore it without making any attempt to change it. Ultimately, you'll want to practice this exercise on the fly, in the midst of your daily activities at work or home. See if you can keep your attention focused on just noticing your emotions in the midst of distractions. This is a very important skill for managing stressful situations, as emotions themselves can pull your attention in all sorts of unproductive directions.

Practice: Watching Thoughts

As we've mentioned, thinking can often create more stress than external stressors do. Yet most people find it much more difficult to watch their thinking than to attend to their senses or shift focus from internal to external stimuli. For this reason, we recommend that you practice the previous exercises until they become familiar and easier before moving on to thought watching.

Whereas emotions tend to show up as visceral reactions in your body, thoughts appear as words in your mind's eye. A good way to observe thoughts is to treat them as words that are written on the pages of a book. When a thought shows up in your mind's eye, imagine putting it on a blank page in your imaginary book. Sometimes it pays to say the thoughts you're observing out loud, as this converts them into something tangible; or you can actually write the thoughts on a piece of paper.

Practice: Observing with Soft Eyes

The practice of soft eyes involves paying attention in a flexible, accepting way to whatever comes into your consciousness. Like thought watching, it can be a bit more challenging than the earlier exercises, in this case because you'll be applying your growing observer abilities in less controlled contexts.

To practice, integrate soft eyes into your ongoing daily activities on several planned occasions each week. An example might be taking a walk during a work break, an activity that offers an abundance of opportunities for practice. While walking, notice whatever catches your eye and gently focus your attention on its details, such as the color of a leaf or the fragile structure of a bud. See if you can just get present with the fact that this is you paying attention to whatever you're paying attention to. This simple observing skill can be applied to any number of activities, such as looking at art, listening to music that you enjoy, playing with your kids, or interacting with a pet. There are opportunities for practicing soft eyes everywhere in daily life. We encourage you to practice it often. It's a great way to get in contact with the moment-by-moment experience of being alive!

Practice: Being a Social Observer

Adopting the observer stance in social contexts tends to be a slightly more difficult skill to master. When it comes to interactions with friends, family, children, or coworkers, we're conditioned to function in participant mode. Nevertheless, people watching is an extremely valuable observing skill that you can practice in fun and playful ways, and it will be immensely helpful if your stress tends to be related to interpersonal conflicts. The goal is to learn to shift attention between internal events (emotions, thoughts, memories, or sensations) triggered by social interactions and the social context surrounding you (facial expressions, tone of voice and loudness, gestures, and so on).

We recommend practicing this skill while engaged in everyday activities, such as going to the park with your child, shopping for groceries, participating in a work meeting, or attending a class. To ensure you practice, plan in advance for a few occasions when you'll do so. Of course, it's fine to practice in unplanned situations as well. Within the social interaction, allow your attention to shift naturally between your internal reactions and the external social context. Throughout, your job is to experience simple awareness (the observer perspective) and allow whatever happens to happen, knowing that you can choose to change your level of participation as the social context changes. For example, you might choose to maintain the observer perspective when stressful thoughts, feelings, or sensations arise, but you might adopt the participant stance when your child falls off a swing and needs to be comforted. As soon as you complete any task that requires the participant stance, return to simple awareness of both internal and external events related to the social context. Initially, we recommend that you limit your practice time to ten minutes or less, and then increase your practice time as you feel comfortable doing so.

Practice Makes Permanent

In this section, we'll help you write out your commitment to practicing the exercises in this chapter. Practicing observer skills formally, via exercises, will help you to live your day-to-day life with more awareness and a greater ability to intentionally shift your focus of attention. You can train your nervous system to shift into parasympathetic mode (quiet mind) often, so the sympathetic nervous system is activated less often, and generally only when necessary. Take a moment to plan your practice by considering the following questions and writing your responses in your journal:

- What brain training practices or exercises do you plan to use?

- When will you practice? Be specific: note the date and time of day for planned practices.

- Who will be your ally in practice, and what type of support will you request?

- How will you celebrate your first week of practice?

Gentle Reminders

Being an observer involves being able to both focus and flexibly shift your attention based upon the demands of the situation you're in. This is a key skill for increasing your ability to function under stress. Stress tends to impair attention, making it narrowly focused, unstable, and biased toward negative information while ignoring positive information. When you can't focus your attention and stay in the role of an observer of your reactions, you become absorbed by negative emotions. You'll feel like there's no way to escape from or solve the problems that are producing stress. The flexible, highly focused attention cultivated by the exercises in this chapter will help you regulate your physical and emotional reactions to stress and solve problems in an efficient, effective way. Regularly practicing these brain training techniques will help you access this focused yet flexible attention on command.

Adopting an observer stance with respect to your stress reactions will put you in good position to describe your reactions in a more objective, accurate way. This is the next skill you'll need to acquire in your five-step program to transcend stress, so read on!

CHAPTER 5

Describe

Without knowing the force of words, it is impossible to know more.

—Confucius

To transcend daily stress, you must be able to recognize, process, and regulate the immediate and sometimes powerful reactions stress can trigger. Stress can inhibit your ability to use language to describe your experience in a way that allows you access the resources of quiet mind. This is because most stress reactions are bundled in such a way as to produce an overwhelming array of physical sensations, memories, and emotions within a matter of seconds. Using words to describe your immediate experience helps you unpack these components of the stress reaction so that you can talk about them individually. This will help you slow down the cascade of stress symptoms, allowing you to process each one and be much more deliberate in your responses.

If you lack describing skills, you're more vulnerable to getting absorbed in stress reactions rather than optimally addressing the problems that create them. This can lead to using words in ways that will only make things worse. Your stress management tool kit needs to include language skills that will help you calm the emotional storm within, activate quiet mind, and respond effectively. This doesn't mean you can or should try to eliminate evaluative thoughts and negative feeling states, such as anger and fear. However, you can learn to use words to help you deal with them more skillfully.

In this chapter, you'll learn powerful strategies that will help you be aware of your stress reactions without becoming embroiled in them. First you'll learn skills for identifying and describing your immediate responses to stress—including feelings, thoughts, sensations, and memories—in the moment, as they arise. Then we'll teach you how to avoid engaging in hidden, counterproductive judgments of your reactions. If such judgments are left unchecked, they'll trigger urges to avoid or escape difficult emotions, tying up your brain's resources.

Words can help you organize and make sense of what you're experiencing. By linking words with various aspects of your internal experience, such as emotions, memories, sensations, and evaluations, you can slow the pace of those experiences and make better sense of what you're feeling or thinking. The process of describing both stress and inner experience is central to success in dealing with everyday challenges—so much so that well-worn clichés address the helplessness that arises when an experience is so extreme that it cannot be put into words: "That insult left me speechless." "I couldn't get a word out of my mouth." "There are no words to describe how hurt I was."

Core Describing Skills

In this chapter, we'll discuss the two core features of describing and provide exercises for practicing both. The first is the ability to use a wide spectrum of words to identify various types and gradations of your immediate responses to stress and the wide variety of mental events that follow. Having ready access to words that describe your initial response to stress and the mental experiences that follow can help you transcend stress and respond more flexibly.

To give you an idea of the power of word choices, read the following words and notice your response: "horrible," "terrible," and "intolerable." Compare that response with the images, thoughts, and feelings these words evoke: "unanticipated," "unfortunate," and "challenging." Descriptive responses to stress tend to elicit responses more aligned with quiet mind, even when the stress itself evokes avoidance. Similarly, descriptive responses to thoughts and feelings tend to promote more calm and a greater sense of confidence than highly evaluative terms.

Consider the example of a woman responding to her experience of sadness when watching a movie that reminds her of her loss of a good friend in a car crash. She could describe her response in any of the following ways: "I'll never get over this," "I hate this stupid movie," "I hate my life; it will never be good again," or "This hurts my heart. I'm crying now. I loved my friend so much, and I miss him every day." The first three responses would amp up restless mind and fuel avoidance, while the last one would promote a sense of acceptance and resolution of her emotional experience of loss.

The second core feature of describing is the ability to describe non-judgmentally. This means not inserting evaluations or mental rules about stress reactions into your immediate processing of them. When negative evaluations are inserted as if they're facts, they tend to trigger unworkable attempts to avoid, escape, or suppress feelings. In the previous example, a description such as "I'm so messed up; I should be over this" would only add to the distress of the experience. If you view feeling sad as being a bad thing, then you're much more likely to try to escape or suppress sadness.

There's a natural tendency to try to avoid stressful situations. Sometimes that works, and sometimes it doesn't. When we can't avoid a stressful situation, we need to have skills that help us turn to face it and honor the feelings and emotions the stress evokes. Describing is a core skill for transcending stress in these circumstances.

Know Your Stress Processing Style

Everyone has a unique way of approaching and processing the emotional reactions that stress produces. These processing styles have three main components: evaluating the feeling tone of the experience, knowing your response tendencies, and being aware of judgment biases you might be susceptible to. How you work with and handle each of these components can make a big difference in how you respond to daily stress. As we discuss these three qualities below, we'll outline strategies for working with each one most effectively. But overall, the key is to be very clear about your stress processing style so you can efficiently recognize and integrate your reactions to stress in a healthy way.

A crucial strategy is to step back from your immediate response, pause, and then describe the *feeling tone* of your stress response as it comes into your awareness. As mentioned earlier, your brain is hardwired to immediately identify the threat level of whatever you focus your attention on. Within milliseconds of zeroing in on a stress reaction, the arousal and calming circuitries of your brain (the sympathetic and parasympathetic nervous systems, respectively) are interacting to determine the level of arousal needed to respond optimally. Simply put, your knee-jerk reaction to a new experience can quickly determine which part of your nervous system gets activated. How do you categorize the stressor? Is it pleasant, unpleasant, or neutral? An unpleasant feeling tone is likely to activate more negative emotions within you and prepare you for some type of action, whereas a positive or neutral feeling tone is likely to activate calming circuitry that promotes reflection and incorporation of more information when determining a response.

Thus, the first strategy to apply when confronting a stressful experience is to pause and see what's pulling you toward becoming aroused rather than remaining calm. The more deliberate you can be in reviewing your feelings, the more likely it is that you'll activate the calming circuitry of the PNS. What are your reactions telling you about the situation you're in? Can you use this information to help you adjust course and try something different? Try using your immediate responses to cue you to use descriptive language to further define your experience and choose how to respond.

A second strategy is to understand your response tendencies when certain kinds of stressful experiences show up. A *response tendency* is an urge to act in a certain way in a particular type of situation. Do you tend to approach certain types of situations and, with others, shift into reverse and get the heck away from them? Generally, unwillingness to approach a particular type of unpleasant stress (for example, criticism) in combination with a tendency to evaluate your worth (or the worth of the person criticizing you) adds to the intensity and negativity of the experience.

For most people, this most typically occurs in the context of work life; but it may also happen in family life. For example, you might choose not to talk to your child when he's playing a zombie video game because you don't like the violent tone of zombie games and don't like to be in the room when that unpleasant emotional tone is present. But one result might be that you lose opportunities to form a stronger relationship with your child in the context of a fairly frequent activity. Every response tendency has an upside and a downside to it, even in the context of positive experiences. The key is to be aware of your response tendencies and understand their risks and benefits in any particular situation.

A third strategy is to be aware of *judgmental biases* about your stress reactions. These are rather automatic appraisals that the mind is prone to make when a complicated or difficult stress response is triggered, regardless of the context in which you have that reaction. For example, you might try to suppress or avoid anger associated with a provocative remark from a challenging family member. This might be due to a judgment bias that because anger feels bad, it's harmful. However, this ignores the fact that there might be situations where getting a little angry could be helpful, such as when you need to call up energy to try out a more assertive response to a somewhat reckless family member. In such situations, anger can motivate you to learn new skills and prepare to perform them well.

Getting tangled up in automatic evaluations (for example, "Only inferior people feel angry" or "Anger proves you're messed up and out of control") amplifies the stress associated with the emotion and makes it harder to work with. In contrast, learning to stay with objective descriptions of your experience (for example, "I'm feeling angry when I have the thought of a holiday dinner with my uncle Don") may help you better access quiet mind. In this way, you can utilize the information contained in a stress response (and in recurring stress-provoking situations) to help you choose a more effective response.

The Witness Perspective

A good way to approach describing skills is to imagine that you're on the witness stand in a courtroom. The job of the witness is to simply report on what was seen without elaborating on it or inserting personal reactions into the testimony. As the witness, your job is to report only what you know from firsthand experience without offering your interpretations of events. Any deviation from being objective makes your testimony less useful. So in order to be a good witness, you must not only be a good observer but also be good at using language that's mostly free from hidden evaluations.

Therefore, when you work on describing your experience directly, your goal is to stay with the facts as you directly observe them. For example, you might be watching a movie that evokes painful memories of a friend you've lost contact with. To describe your experience directly you might say, "I'm having memories of my friend right now. I'm feeling sad and have a lump in my throat." When you deviate from the witness perspective, you might start judging how you're reacting instead of simply being aware of your reactions. For example, "I should be over this. I shouldn't be sad because I actually have a lot to feel happy about in my life."

The Neuroscience of Describing

The field of affective neuroscience is shining new light on how human beings experience and process stress-related emotions at the level of brain circuitry. Once the structures of the midbrain are activated to produce an immediate response, two distinct brain pathways are activated to help us recognize the potential stressor and interpret its meaning. The first pathway involves the simple recognition that a stressor is present and a response is needed. This orienting response helps you decide if the stressor is positive, negative, or neutral.

The second pathway involves more in-depth evaluation or cognitive appraisal, including the degree of danger or threat—or, alternatively, the degree of pleasure. This more in-depth evaluation may produce a flood of emotional responses, thoughts, memories, and sensations, from *I love chocolate cake* to *He's being mean to me on purpose.* The brain and mind then work together to figure out the potential usefulness of emotions in guiding behavioral responses, such as cutting a large piece of cake for yourself or giving someone an angry look. Emotion is integral to this second, and more critical, pathway, in which a cognitive appraisal fleshes out your preparatory response to the stressor. This immediately prepares your nervous system to help you approach, avoid, attack, or collapse.

If you get absorbed in a negative appraisal, like telling yourself that feeling angry isn't okay because you should be positive, this actually results in more negative, intense, and intrusive responses to stress because the neural circuitry responsible for exerting a calming influence isn't being activated. This leaves the limbic system in a state of ongoing arousal. As a result, restless mind continues to scan for negative information (which it can easily find), so your stress responses continue to escalate.

The alternative is to stay nonjudgmental, not assigning highly negative appraisals to your descriptions of stressors and your stress response, whether that response is characterized by negative or positive thoughts, emotions, or physical sensations. Taking the nonjudgmental perspective that these experiences are what they are and nothing more triggers PNS activation, which in turn reduces activity of the arousal centers in the limbic system. The result is that you move from restless mind arousal to a state of quiet mind. And only in a state of quiet mind can you really understand your reactions to stress-producing experiences and choose how to respond.

The Neuroscience of Describing

The core skills involved in describing, the underlying neural circuits, and the associated mental processes are outlined below.

Describing skill: Recognizing and naming stressors and emotional states

Areas of the brain involved

- Anterior cingulate nucleus

- Medial orbitofrontal cortex

Mental processes

- Discriminating the affective tone of a private experience

- Activating arousal regulation functions

Describing skill: Remaining nonjudgmental

Areas of the brain involved

- Ventrolateral prefrontal cortex

- Dorsal anterior cingulate nucleus

Mental processes

- Allowing nonreactive cognitive appraisal of affective tone

- Reducing physiological arousal associated with emotions

- Strengthening self-regulation of emotion-based behavior

Brain Training

In this section, we offer some simple practices that will help you become more skillful in describing stressors and using your powers of description to accept your thoughts, physical sensations, and especially your emotions in stressful circumstances. We want to help you stop fighting your emotions and instead use them to guide you—after you've processed them in a state of quiet mind.

Exercise: Describing Daily Hassles and Your Response to Them

This exercise will help you learn to better describe your daily hassles and your emotional responses to them. You'll find a downloadable worksheet for this purpose at http://www.newharbinger.com/31274 (see the back of this book for instructions on how to access it). Alternatively, you can create a similar form, perhaps in your journal for this book, using the four columns in the downloadable worksheet: "Daily hassle" on the left, then "Feeling tone," then "Response tendency," and finally "Emotional response" on the right.

To do the exercise, choose a recent stressful event, perhaps from your Daily Hassles and Helpers Log, and examine it using the following process:

1. In the left-hand column, describe the daily hassle using the witness perspective and descriptive language.

2. Check your feeling tone. Using cues in your body and mental experiences, determine whether the feeling tone is pleasant, unpleasant, or neutral.

3. Continue to notice your mind and body and assess your response tendency. Do you have an inclination to approach, ignore, or avoid your experience?

4. Shift your focus to your emotional experience. Are you sad, mad, glad, fearful, guilty, excited, or happy, or are you experiencing some other emotion?

Continue practicing this exercise with a broad range of daily hassles, whatever form they may take: hearing an incessantly barking dog, waiting in a long line, feeling hungry, and so on. This will improve your ability to describe your emotional state and, ultimately, help you access quiet mind.

Exercise: Reeling in Evaluations Gone Wild

Brain training is all about becoming more flexible in responding to stressful situations. This exercise will help you become more familiar with the evaluations your mind tries to inject into stressful situations. When these evaluations go undetected, your responses become more automatic and inflexible. As discussed in the neuroscience section, objective descriptions produce dramatically different results at the brain circuitry level than evaluations do, so it's crucial to develop your ability to distinguish between these two types of thinking.

You'll find a downloadable worksheet for this exercise at http://www.newharbinger.com/31274. Alternatively, you can create a similar form, perhaps in your journal for this book, using the three columns in the downloadable worksheet: "Stressful situation" on the left, "Witness perspective" in the center, and "Evaluations gone wild" on the right.

Select three or four stressors for your practice session and, for each, examine it using the following process:

1. Briefly note the nature of the stressor in the left-hand column; for example, "A loud noise."

2. In the middle column, write a brief description of your experience with the stressful situation from the witness perspective. Challenge

yourself to use only objective descriptions; for example, "The noise was loud. When I first heard it, I covered my ears."

3. Finally, practice being as judgmental and evaluative as possible about the same event, then write your evaluations in the right-hand column. Don't hold back! Let your mind's evaluative functions run wild; for example, "The noise was horrible. It was painful and piercing and I thought it would puncture my eardrums." It's okay to have some fun with the evaluations and make them outlandish.

Practice: Describing Your Inner Experience

In this exercise, you'll get more experience in objectively describing your inner experiences, such as thoughts, emotions, memories, or physical sensations. To begin, find an internal physical sensation to focus on: your heartbeat, your breath, or any other sensation in your body that comes into your awareness. Fix your attention on that focus point.

Next, begin describing what shows up for you once your attention is fixed on the focus point. It may take a minute or two, but soon you'll begin to notice various internal experiences showing up in your awareness. The goal is to describe them on a moment-to-moment basis using all of the words you have at your disposal. The best way is to simply name what's showing up in your experience; for example, "I feel tingling in my hands," "I'm having the thought that my boss doesn't like me," "I'm aware of the feeling called guilty," "I'm aware of a smile emerging on my face," "I'm having the feeling called curiosity," "I'm aware of feeling sad," "I'm having worrisome thoughts about something being wrong with my children," "I'm aware of a choking sensation is my throat and pressure in my chest," and so on.

The goal is to simply describe what's present in your internal world and direct moment-to-moment experience without judging or evaluating it. You don't have to figure out why you're feeling sad or worried or whether you should or shouldn't be having a certain feeling or thought. At this point, it isn't important to understand where your experience comes from.

As you practice, notice and describe what happens next. In particular, does your overall level of awareness change or stay the same? It's best to practice several times over the course of your day (for example, morning, noon, and evening). Also, it's fine if your practice periods are brief; three to five minutes is enough.

As you get more comfortable using inner witnessing skills, you can begin to extend your use of this exercise, practicing it when you're experiencing a stressful event or engaging in a daily review of stressful events. At some predetermined time, preferably later in the day, such as before dinner or at bedtime, review the stresses of your day and intentionally apply the witness perspective to them. As you bring up each stressful situation, also apply the approach from the first exercise in this chapter, observing the feeling tone and reviewing any urges to act on your feelings. Also note any evaluations you have about whatever emotions you experience.

Practice: Naming Basic Emotions

Being more skillful in describing your emotions will help you better monitor and control your level of arousal. When you're able to detect emotions at lower intensity levels, you increase your ability to use them to inform your responses to stress. Basic emotions include feeling sad, mad, glad, and afraid. For this exercise, practice using these simple words to describe your varying emotions. We recommend that you practice for an hour or two per week, and that you schedule times for doing so one or two days over the next week. Decide on your practice times and set an alarm on your phone or watch to provide a reminder. During that time period, repeat the following process every time you notice an emotion arising:

1. Briefly note the basic emotion name: sad, mad, glad, or afraid.

2. Rate the level of intensity of the emotion using a scale of 1 to 10, where 1 is very low intensity and 10 is very high intensity.

3. Continue watching the emotion and rating it every thirty to sixty seconds to track changes in intensity. You may find that taking a few slow, deep breaths improves your focus, allowing you to detect and describe changes in emotions and their intensity.

Exercise: Making Descriptive Requests

Many stressors occur in the context of relating to other people. For example, you may have a difference of opinion with a coworker, or you may feel frustrated by your child's problematic behavior. This exercise will help you develop skill in using descriptive phrases to express what you want or need from others.

You'll find a downloadable worksheet for this exercise at http://www.newharbinger.com/31274. Alternatively, you can create a similar form, perhaps in your journal for this book, using the three columns in the downloadable worksheet: "Interpersonal stress" on the left, "Desired outcome" in the center, and "Descriptive request" on the right.

Select three or four interpersonal stressors for your practice session and, for each, examine it using the following process:

1. Briefly note the nature of the stressor in the left-hand column; for example, "My boss asks me to work late."

2. In the middle column, write a brief description of your desired outcome, based on your response to the stressor. Challenge yourself to use only objective descriptions; for example, "As I leave, my boss smiles and thanks me for staying thirty minutes late to help out."

3. Finally, write the phrase you would like to use to create the outcome you desire; for example, "I'm willing to stay thirty minutes if you'd find that helpful. What do you think?"

Practice Makes Permanent

In this section, we'll help you write out your commitment to practicing some of the exercises in this chapter. Routinely practicing describing skills will help you to use them in the heat of the moment, when your stress level is high. The more often you practice, the more you'll strengthen the neural circuits that help you regulate stress-related emotions. This, in turn, will help you activate quiet mind, so daily practice is recommended. Take a moment to plan your practice by considering the following questions and writing your responses in your journal:

- What brain training practices or exercises do you plan to use?

- When will you practice? Be specific: note the date and time of day for planned practices.

- Who will be your ally in practice, and what type of support will you request?

- How will you celebrate your first week of practice?

Gentle Reminders

A key mindfulness strategy for transcending stress is developing your powers of description so you can use words to help you both understand and control your reactions to stressful experiences. Taking a witness perspective involves being able to describe your stress responses without unnecessary negativity.

There are three key strategies that will help you approach your stress responses nonjudgmentally: using descriptive terms to define the stressor, noticing the feeling tone of your response, and being aware of your patterns of evaluation and action as they arise in the moment. You can gain the upper hand over your reactions to stress and be more effective in how you respond if you're willing to stay in contact with inner experiences, even if they're unpleasant, and use words to help you describe those experiences.

Adopting the witness perspective with your stress responses will put you in a good position to practice detachment from restless mind's negative evaluations. This is the next skill you'll need to acquire in your five-step program to transcend stress, so read on!

CHAPTER 6

Detach

He who would be serene and pure needs but one thing: detachment.

—Meister Eckhart

Detachment is a key mindfulness skill that will help you reduce the problematic impacts of daily stress. Stress tends to overactivate restless mind, and if you overidentify with your stressors and stress reactions, they'll seem much more dangerous to your well-being. This dramatically increases the chance that you'll respond impulsively and ineffectively.

Detachment is the antidote for the problem of overidentifying with restless mind, as it allows you to respond mindfully to stress and minimize your use of escape, avoidance, or confrontation strategies. By learning to take a detached stance in which you step back and just allow your thoughts and feelings to be there, you'll increase your ability to respond to stress in more transcendent ways. After all, these are just your reactions to a temporary life challenge, and you are not the same as your reactions. Rather, you are the person who is aware of your reactions. Detachment involves anchoring your awareness in the important distinction between you and your immediate reactions.

In this chapter, we'll teach you how to step back and create some space between yourself and your thoughts, emotions, memories, and physical sensations. From this perspective, there's no compelling need to struggle with your reactions or allow them to determine your behavior. Instead, you can allow your reactions to be present while focusing your attention on what matters to you in the moment.

Stress responses may appear when you're about to engage in something that's important to you, like approaching an argument with your spouse or partner in a healthy way even though your feelings are hurt. If you take hurt feelings to heart or identify with them, they might lead you to be more aggressive toward your partner than you wish to be. However, if you take perspective on your hurt feelings and see them as no real threat to your welfare, even though they're painful, you can focus your attention on conducting yourself in a way that's true to your principles in regard to being an intimate partner.

Detachment doesn't mean you necessarily like being in the presence of stressful inner (and outer) experiences; it simply means you're willing to make room for them. In this state, you can see stresses in a more objective way, experience emotions with acceptance, see thoughts and memories as products of the mind, and look at sensations with curiosity. You can use your attention wisely as you work with stresses through the day and be a human experiencing daily hassles without letting those hassles dominate your attention.

Core Detachment Skills

We'll focus on two central features of detachment in this chapter. First, detachment involves accepting what's present in your awareness, knowing that it need not be controlled in any way—and probably can't be controlled anyway. In the midst of a stress reaction, you simply recognize what's there, seeing it for what it is (an unpleasant thought, feeling, memory, or sensation), not what restless mind says it is (a threat to your personal well-being). Second, detachment requires that you step back from whatever is there and take a long view of the stress-producing situation. This allows you to see that what seems important today is (usually) just small stuff. As powerful as the emotions of the moment are, the situation doesn't warrant overriding your life principles or chosen direction. This is sometimes called taking the eagle perspective.

The Eagle Perspective

When you attach to a mental experience like a negative thought, emotion, or memory, you become part of the experience you're attached to, leaving you with a shortsighted perspective. In this state, your responses are likely to be guided by self-protective motives, such as being in control, being right, getting revenge, treating someone unfairly to show them how it feels to be you, and so on. Of course, these aren't lofty human goals, and even if you achieve them, you won't feel better about yourself in the long run.

On the other side of the coin is the eagle perspective, which allows you to see your current stress in the big picture of your life. Seen from this detached perspective, very few stressful situations or interactions are worth fighting over, feeling victimized about, or seeking revenge for. In a state of attachment, being passed over for a promotion you feel you deserve might seem like the end of the world and extremely unfair, and you may feel that someone needs to be punished for the mistake. The eagle perspective is that not getting the promotion opens different doors for you, and that five years from now you might see this same event as a major positive turning point in your life. Things that are a big deal when you have an attached, shortsighted perspective on daily life cease to be meaningful from this more nuanced view. The famous saying by Richard Carlson (1997)—also the title of his book—makes the point better than we can: Don't sweat the small stuff….and it's all small stuff!

Nonjudgmental absorption and awe—meaning the ability to detach oneself from the world and the burden of painful emotions like loss or anxiety—are definitive features of what Abraham Maslow called peak experience (1964). A *peak experience* is a moment when the whole of life and the universe is seen from a new, detached, and compassionate point of view. When you free yourself from your own mind, you're likely to find that what shows up in that void is worth waiting around for! While there are no guarantees in life, actively practicing detachment skills will bring you closer to peak experiences and special moments in whatever venue makes the most sense to you, spiritually or otherwise. It might turn out that simply observing a stunning sunset is a great way for you to explore the life-altering benefits of detachment. Here's a thought to ponder at your next sunset: You and the sun are moving across the universe in exactly the same direction, at about fifty-two thousand miles per hour!

The Neuroscience of Detachment

Within microseconds of making contact with a stressful stimulus, areas of the primitive brain are activated that allow us to orient to the stimulus, sort it into general emotional categories (pleasant, neutral, or unpleasant), and generate an evaluation of the relevance of the stimulus: *How important is this? Is it a threat? Is it an opportunity? Am I up to it? Should I fight, freeze, or run?*

Whereas the task of orienting, sorting, and conducting an initial threat assessment lies within the neural circuitry of the SNS, the task of *reappraisal* lies in the advanced arousal-regulating structures of the prefrontal cortex (Ochsner and Gross 2008; Schuyler et al. 2012). Activation of these structures triggers the PNS to put the brakes on premature emotional arousal prior to completion of the more complex neural task of appraisal, which necessarily involves activation of several specific areas of the forebrain.

There are two basic neural pathways involved in appraisal. One supports conscious verbal attempts to reduce estimates of threat (for example, "Anyone would be upset about being passed over for a job promotion they thought they deserved, and it isn't the end of the world if my feelings are hurt"). The goal of conscious verbal reappraisal is to "talk yourself down" and thus regulate the intensity of stress responses. With this type of appraisal, it typically takes longer to achieve a reduction in SNS arousal.

The second, and more intriguing, neural pathway is activated when the process of appraisal involves adjusting the personal relevance of the stressor and the response it evokes. Stress responses are simply observed without attachment to meanings generated by the mind. There is no effort to sort through the meanings or evaluate them; the effort is in letting the responses come and go of their own accord. Interestingly, this type of appraisal acts very quickly to reduce SNS arousal.

Taking a detached stance has been shown to reduce various markers of SNS arousal in response to a distressing emotional experience (Kalisch et al. 2005). SNS activation affects the cardiovascular system in surprisingly specific ways. For example, blood flow to major muscle groups increases. With the emotion of anger, blood flow increases to the arms (preparing for a fight), and with fear, blood flows more powerfully to the legs (preparing to run). Breathing also changes as stress increases: we tend to hold our breath, extracting as much oxygen as possible from every inhalation. In addition, norepinephrine and epinephrine surge throughout the body, impacting multiple systems, with increased norepinephrine priming the brain for activation.

The bottom line is, without the aid of detachment, you'll eventually be able to put the brakes on the harmful biochemical impacts of the SNS by talking yourself down, but it can take quite a bit longer to activate your PNS. And you might instead end up "talking yourself up," becoming even more physiologically aroused, because trying to change your evaluations of a situation or interaction can be very tricky when you're emotionally aroused. Thus, detachment isn't just useful for protecting yourself in extreme circumstances; it's also a core lifestyle skill for moderating the harmful mental and physical effects of prolonged exposure to daily stress.

The Neuroscience of Detaching

The core skills involved in detachment, the underlying neural circuits, and the associated mental processes are outlined below.

Detachment skill: Acceptance of emotion without the need to react (having a sense of limited personal relevance)

Areas of the brain involved

- Medial prefrontal cortex
- Anterior cingulate cortex

Mental processes

- Decreasing SNS activation
- Decreasing the perceived relevance of distressing private experiences

Detachment skill: Self-related perspective taking

Areas of the brain involved

- Anterolateral prefrontal cortex

Mental processes

- Supporting representation of the self as distinct from the object of attention
- Reducing emotional arousal through cognitive reappraisal

Brain Training

In this section, you'll learn several brain training exercises that will help you strengthen your detachment skills. Most of these strategies are easy to practice within the typical flow of daily life. For those that require setting aside time to practice, we'll give you an estimate of the amount of time you'll need to carve out of your daily schedule.

Practice: Belly Breathing

Practicing deep, even breathing, often called *belly breathing*, can foster quiet mind and is important for developing a detached perspective. It clears the effects of SNS activation from your mind so you can reexamine and take perspective on the stressful situation you're facing.

To experience the muscles involved in belly breathing, lie on your stomach and take a slow, deep breath. You'll notice your belly pressing into the floor. As you breathe out, contract the same muscles you'd use to do a sit-up. Your ribs and pelvis will move toward the floor. Tuning in to these sensations will help you get a feel for belly breathing. When you're familiar with these sensations, try belly breathing while lying on your back or sitting. Place the palm of one hand on your belly to provide the same kind of feedback the floor provides when you're lying on your stomach.

Practice four or five cycles of belly breathing four or five times per day to reset your nervous system and develop facility in detaching from stressful emotions. You might want to use various daily activities as cues for breathing practice, such as sitting down to eat a meal, waiting at a red light, or ending a phone call. There are a variety of smartphone applications that provide visual aids for belly breathing, and you may want to try using some of them to support your practice. Once you become familiar with belly breathing, try using this technique anytime you feel stressed-out. You'll probably be amazed at how calming it is.

Practice: Separating Speaker and Listener

The simplest way to practice detachment is to change how you describe the relationship between you and your mind. Remember, you are the human being, and your mind is a creation of the brain that speaks to you. The mind is a speaker, and you, the human, are a listener. One way to train your brain to create space between speaker and listener is by deliberately changing how you talk about this relationship.

Cubbyholing

One fun way to practice separating the speaker and the listener is to simply label or categorize whatever comes up in your attention, for example, "thought...feeling...thought...memory...sensation ...thought...memory..." This type of exercise is called *cubbyholing* because you take each type of mental product and place it in the appropriate cubbyhole. All the memories go into one cubbyhole, all the thoughts go into another, all the emotions go into the emotions cubbyhole, and so forth.

This exercise increases your awareness of and ability to discriminate between different kinds of mental products. It also teaches you to respond to the *type* of product your mind is giving you, rather than the message that product contains. For example, a memory of a painful interpersonal rejection goes in the same cubbyhole as a memory of a peak experience on a camping trip. You can say the categories out loud if you like; just watch out if people are around, and make sure they know what you're up to! Alternatively, you can state the categories silently to yourself. You can also use simple sentences if you like, such as "There's a thought" or "That's a memory."

Labeling Internal Experiences

Another thing you can try is creating sentences that acknowledge your experience of what your mind is presenting (Hayes, Strosahl, and Wilson 1999; Strosahl and Robinson 2008). For example, instead of saying, "I'm pissed off about not getting a raise at work," you could say, "I'm having the thought that I'm pissed off about not getting a raise" or "I'm aware of the emotion of anger about not getting a raise." Practicing this way of talking, which highlights the distinction between speaker (the mind) and listener (the self), allows you to take the perspective of the human being who is aware of these experiences. Several variations on this basic strategy are possible. In addition to the stem phrases "I'm aware of [thought, feeling, memory, sensation]..." and "I'm having the [thought, feeling, memory, sensation]...," you could also say "I'm noticing the [thought, feeling, memory, sensation]..." or "What just showed up is the [thought, emotion, memory, sensation] called..."

Exercise: Working with Flypaper Experiences

Some aspects of a stress response are harder to detach from than others, and no one is immune to getting hooked by highly provocative thoughts or emotions, such as being right when someone else is wrong, evaluating an emotional reaction as bad, thinking you're being screwed by life, or blaming yourself for making a mistake or letting someone down. A name we use for these dark moments is "flypaper experiences." If you aren't familiar with flypaper, it's a simple, effective way to trap and kill houseflies: thin strips of paper covered with a sweet syrup that flies can't resist, which you hang from the ceiling. When flies land on the paper, they stick to the syrup and can't escape.

In a similar way, once you land on seemingly important but ultimately self-defeating stress reactions, you can't lift off and separate from them, no matter how hard you try. When this happens, your level of suffering immediately increases. Given that these experiences are inevitable, it's best to openly acknowledge them and examine them in a way that's lighthearted and doesn't involve you attempting to control them.

In this exercise, you'll put your flypaper thoughts, feelings, memories, and sensations out in the open. First, get a pad of sticky notes and write down one flypaper experience per sticky note (for example, "I'm not there enough for my kids"). Normally, if you're feeling stressed by a particular life situation, you'll have a number of sticky notes describing various thoughts, feelings, memories, and physical symptoms associated with that situation. You can randomly stick these notes all over your body, or you can organize them by type (for example, all the memories on your left shoulder). Then, spend ten minutes or so walking around with these flypaper experiences, periodically reading each one out loud and then sticking it back on. You can even have other people look at the sticky notes and read them to you. This is the ultimate in detachment: allowing others to see your dirty laundry while you practice maintaining eagle perspective!

Practice: Thanking Your Mind

A great way to practice detachment from flypaper experiences is to thank your mind out loud for giving you a disturbing thought, distressing emotion, or painful memory. This reminds you that there's a difference between you, the human, and the mind that's chattering at you. For example, you might say, "Thank you, mind, for giving me a heads-up about my flaws as a parent (or student, or employee). You're doing your job, and I'm aware of your input." Anytime you notice that you've suddenly attached to something painful, you can extract yourself by immediately thanking your mind for giving you the painful experience.

If you notice that a certain stress-related emotion, thought, or memory repeatedly functions like flypaper for you, you can write a gratitude statement for it on several sticky notes and post those notes where you'll see them on a daily basis, such as on the dashboard of your car or your bathroom mirror. It's good to shift the location of these written reminders from week to week so you'll continue to notice them. You could even come up with new expressions of gratitude each week; for example, one week you might write, "Hey, brain buddy, way to go on warning me that I'm not as smart as my coworkers! I'm sure glad you're on the job!" Then, the next week, you could come up with a different statement, such as "Thanks, mind, for reminding me that my hairline is receding and everyone must surely notice that as their first impression of me. I'll keep that in mind as I continue to make friends."

Practice: Seeing the Mind as an Internal Advisor

This exercise allows you to zero in on your mind's typical ways of advising you about stress so you're less likely to be caught off guard. For several days, check in with yourself whenever a significant stressful event happens and ask yourself, "What is my mind telling me about this?" We recommend that you write out your mind's advice—which is usually to take a shortsighted view and overreact—and then review it from time to time so you can recognize it in the moment. This will help promote detachment and quiet-mind experience even amidst advice from restless mind to get busy and run, fight, or hide!

Practice: Watching Clouds in the Sky

If the problem is that certain stressful thoughts, emotions, memories, or sensations trap you like flypaper, then learning not to get stuck to these sticky creatures is the solution! This simple, elegant exercise will help you develop the ability to let go of troublesome thoughts, emotions, memories, and sensations. It requires five to ten minutes of your undivided attention. Find a quiet location where you won't be disturbed and sit or lie down comfortably. (We highly recommend that you try the exercise at least a few times while lying on the grass with real clouds above you.)

Imagine that you're looking up at the sky and see a variety of clouds floating across your field of vision. They come in all sizes and shapes, and no two are alike. As you become aware of a thought entering your awareness, put that thought onto a cloud and let it float along in the sky with the other clouds. As you make contact with an emotion, do the same thing. When a memory shows up, put it on a cloud. If you notice a sensation in your body, put it on a cloud too. Continue doing this for the entire practice session. You'll probably notice your mind trying to direct your attention elsewhere; for example, you may become aware of a thought like *I'm not very good at this exercise, so I guess I'll never* be very good at detachment. When that happens, put *that* thought on a cloud and refocus your attention on the task at hand.

This exercise can take many forms. For example, you might imagine that you're sitting on the bank of a gently flowing creek. When anything pops into your awareness, name it and then visualize putting it on a leaf and watching it slowly float downstream. Or you can imagine that you're stopped at a railroad crossing with a train passing slowly in front you. As you become aware of a thought, feeling, memory, or sensation, name the experience, place it on a boxcar, and then let the boxcar slowly move across your field of vision.

Practice: Generating Opposites

For this exercise, you'll use writing as a way to practice first reacting from an attached perspective and then consciously responding from a detached perspective. Think of a recent stressful situation, notice a judgmental evaluation of it, and let yourself attach to that evaluation. Then write a narrative about the situation. Next, let go of that evaluation and write a second, more detached account.

For example, let's say someone cut you off on the highway. Afterward, explore your interpretations of the event in writing, beginning with a very attached perspective. There's a good chance that if you just let your writing flow and avoid thinking about whether you're attached or detached, the attached perspective will be the first to emerge—for example, "That jerk. What's he trying to do, kill someone? What's wrong with him? He should have his driver's license pulled!" Next, take a detached perspective on that same scenario and write about the event again—for example, "Wow! That was close. I am thankful for my life right now. And I'm glad no one else was hurt."

Do this exercise often, with different situations, to get practice in switching from an attached to a detached perspective. This will help you become familiar with the feeling tones associated with each perspective. You can practice this exercise with almost any type of life event, including positive ones.

Exercise: Mirror, Mirror on the Wall

A quick but challenging way to practice high-level detachment skills is to simply look at yourself in a large or full-length mirror for a prolonged period of time, say five minutes. It's a simple but revealing form of detachment training. If you really want to push the envelope on this exercise, do this without any clothes on, maybe right after taking a bath or shower.

While standing in front of the mirror, first notice any evaluations that show up in your mind's eye; then practice detaching from those evaluations. You might notice historical evaluations starting to appear, comparing how you look now to how you once looked. Maybe the evaluation will be that your appearance today doesn't measure up to your former self. You might notice your mind wandering off into some earlier memory, trying to recall the last time you looked really attractive. Perhaps your mind will start to evaluate your face, finding little flaws for you to get lost in. It may even tell you that you shouldn't be looking at yourself like this—that something bad will happen if you keep looking.

We call this a "bucking bronco" exercise because the mind tends to go crazy when you simply stand and look at yourself. The goal is to use your detachment skills to ride the bucking bronco of the mind no matter what it throws at you. Like a rodeo horse, it will keep trying to throw you off track. Your goal is to call on your detachment skills to adjust to each move the mind makes. If you notice that you got thrown off by attaching to an evaluation, just climb back on and start riding again!

Practice Makes Permanent

In this section, we'll help you write out your commitment to practicing the exercises in this chapter. Regular practice will help you live daily life with both acceptance toward and detachment from whatever is going on, both inside you and in the outside world. It just takes a commitment to practice these exercises on a regular schedule. Most of them can be done while you're in the flow of your daily routine, but a few do require you set aside time to be alone with your mind. Take a moment to plan your practice by considering the following questions and writing your responses in your journal:

- What brain training practices or exercises do you plan to use?

- When will you practice? Be specific: note the date and time of day for planned practices.

- Who will be your ally in practice, and what type of support will you request?

- How will you celebrate your first week of practice?

Gentle Reminders

Detachment is a key mindfulness strategy for transcending stress. It involves accepting stressful emotions, thoughts, memories, and physical sensations with an attitude that they don't pose a threat to you and you don't need to get mentally involved with them. In part, taking a detached stance requires you to establish a relationship with your mind in which it's the speaker and you're the listener. Although you have a mind, you are not the same as your mind! But this important fact often gets obscured in daily living. Detachment allows you to take the eagle perspective on a stressful situation, recognizing that whatever seems important in the moment probably won't be nearly as important in a year. Specific neural pathways in the brain regulate emotional arousal and promote intentional action. Practicing detachment exercises on a regular basis will strengthen these neural connections.

Adopting a detached state of awareness will put you in a good position to take on the most provocative and negative evaluations your mind throws at you: its evaluations of you and your flaws and imperfections. Learning how to relate to your inner critic is the next skill you must acquire in this five-step program to transcend stress, so read on! You're already past the halfway point in your journey.

CHAPTER 7

Love Yourself

Love and compassion are necessities, not luxuries.
Without them, humanity cannot survive.

—Dalai Lama

In this chapter, we'll help you discover that a key step on the path toward transcending stress is to love yourself, warts and all. As you stop taking yourself so seriously, you'll probably find that you aren't that bad after all. The word "self-compassion" is a fitting way to describe the concept of loving yourself. Whatever term you use, kindness toward yourself is a central aspect of mindfulness that can change your entire perspective on what it means to be you and to be alive in this world. Loving yourself is the antidote for every mistake you think you've made, every flaw you think you have, and every disappointment you've endured. And miraculously, loving yourself is absolutely free of charge, and it's available right at your fingertips as you're reading this sentence. Our goal is to help you reach out and grasp it so you can take it with you on your life journey.

Stress has a way of bringing out our imperfections and putting them on display for all to see. Stress might make you irritable and short-tempered with your children, your spouse, or your parents. You might find yourself making excuses so you can avoid a family get-together or night out you'd planned with a friend, and inside, you might start feeling ashamed and guilty about your neglect of family or friends. Your mind's formidable powers might get focused on you as the problem, resulting in a steady stream of negative mental chatter directed your way. Your mind might tell you that you lack something other people have (such as a certain family orientation or loyalty toward friends) or that you have faults (such as being selfish or lazy) that will ultimately ruin your chances of success in life.

Alarmed by this negative inner dialogue, restless mind will shift into high gear and begin scanning for all the flaws you might possibly have (and if you're like us, many will be found!), exaggerating their importance and making you feel like dirt in the process. The only remedy for this dreadful state of affairs is to choose to love yourself with conscious and complete acceptance of your shortcomings. Although taking this unusual step won't get that inner critic off your shoulder, it will put a sock in its mouth so you can at least hear quiet mind reminding you that you're completely lovable just the way you are!

Core Self-Compassion Skills

Practicing self-compassion involves two central features, and we'll focus on both in this chapter. First, it means understanding and accepting the inevitable reality that you will make mistakes, not meet your expectations for yourself, or fail in important life pursuits. A key part of this understanding and acceptance is recognizing that you aren't alone—that everyone has shortcomings. Instead of seeing yourself as flawed and somehow different from everyone else (or perhaps even while receiving that thought from your mind), you can cut yourself some slack and see that you're just like other people. This allows you to let go of the need to be perfect so that you can instead treat yourself with the love and respect that you deserve. In the end, it's okay to be you!

Second, self-compassion requires that you detach from self-defeating personal narratives, however rational and realistic they might appear at first glance. A *personal narrative* is a self-story that explains who you are and how you got to be that way. Personal narratives are one of the basic methods we humans use to try to organize and make sense of the events that mark our life journeys. We also relate to other people by sharing our personal narrative with them (for example, "I'm a person who's good to his word" or "I was an only child, and I've never been as comfortable around other people as I am when I'm by myself").

The Dalai Lama describes this storytelling feature as one of the most destructive aspects of the conceptual mind (2002). It's the mind's attempt to create the appearance of self-understanding, but the problem is, it's only an illusion of self-understanding. Because we use our narratives so much in daily life, we begin to actually believe they're true. When this happens, we become limited in who we are and what we can be in life because we're attached to narratives that put those limitations in place. Therefore, it's important to recognize your self-stories for what they are—stories made up by the mind—rather than the true story of you that they appear to be. Although you can't get rid of restless mind's narratives, you *can* (and will) learn to carry them lightly and use eagle perspective to recognize them for what they are.

The Self-Compassionate Perspective

The journey toward loving yourself starts with some perplexing questions that might have far-reaching implications for your long-term life plan. What if your flaws or shortcomings are as important a part of you as your strengths? What if you *need* shortcomings to understand and be compassionate toward the shortcomings of others? What if accepting your flaws is actually good for your overall health and well-being? What if it's absolutely, positively okay for you (and everyone) to have flaws? Whenever we raise these questions with clients, they typically look down and away, obviously embarrassed to consider these radical ideas. Apparently, we've been trained to believe that it's the height of self-deception to practice such complete acceptance of and love for who we are. That's a pity, because there's a lot to love!

Fortunately, recent research provides good reason to turn this attitude around. In particular, self-compassion plays a critical role in the ability to withstand and transcend stressful life moments. Clinical research has consistently demonstrated that practicing self-compassion has beneficial effects on mental health (Neff 2009). People with high levels of self-compassion tend to be more motivated to learn about themselves, less fixated on gaining the approval of others, and less afraid of making mistakes (Neff, Hsieh, and Dejitterat 2005). Research also suggests that it's possible to develop greater self-compassion by practicing certain skills for a very short period of time. A recent study showed that, after even brief self-compassion training, people had a much more altruistic attitude toward the suffering of others and less difficulty with their own emotions in response to suffering (Weng et al. 2013). Another study showed that a brief self-compassion intervention neutralized the harsh self-criticism that typically leads people on diets to overeat when they violate their diet (Adams and Leary 2007).

The Neuroscience of Self-Compassion

Neuroscience studies have examined the effects of mindfulness practice on both neural structures and processing efficiency in the brain. One exciting finding is that compassion-based mindfulness practice increases the density of gray matter in certain areas of the brain. These areas of the brain are involved in learning and memory processes, as well as emotional control, self-awareness, and perspective taking (Hölzel et al. 2011). Interestingly, social self-awareness (seeing yourself as affiliated with others, which is part of the process of self-compassion) appears to be supported by an overlapping but distinctly different set of neural circuitry associated with empathy and with the ability to mentally visualize and compare different problem-solving approaches (Quirk and Beer 2006).

It also appears that the experience of compassion for oneself and others strengthens neural circuitry responsible for regulating the activity of the amygdala, the brain center involved in producing negative emotions (Schuyler et al. 2012). Therefore, practicing compassion toward yourself or others can help decrease your susceptibility to negative emotional experiences. As discussed, prolonged negative stress-triggered emotions compromise the immune and cardiovascular systems. Thus, there's every reason to believe that practicing self-compassion can also protect your physical health.

The Neuroscience of Self-Compassion

The core skills involved in self-compassion, the underlying neural circuits, and the associated mental processes are outlined below. Due to the complex nature of self-compassion, you'll notice that many different regions of the higher-order brain are involved.

Self-compassion skill: Acceptance and empathy regarding flaws and imperfections in oneself and others

---

Areas of the brain involved

- Left hippocampus

- Posterior cingulate cortex

- Insula

- Temporoparietal junction

- Amygdala

Mental processes

- Activating a prosocial orientation and empathic understanding

- Producing approach-oriented mental responses to the suffering of oneself and others

Self-compassion skill: Perspective taking on narratives or stories about oneself

Areas of the brain involved

- Left dorsal temporoparietal junction

- Precuneus

- Left middle occipital gyrus

Mental processes

- Promoting social perspective taking (I-you)

- Supporting mental representations of different points of view

Brain Training

In this section, we'll give you a variety of brain training exercises designed to increase your self-compassion skills. We encourage you to try all of the exercises and then select a few that really appeal to you to integrate into your brain training regime.

Practice: Engaging a Half-Knowing Smile

The half-knowing smile helps you practice detachment, compassion, and perspective taking all at once. There are numerous other ways to practice this skill, so if you run into alternatives, don't be afraid to try them. The technique is simple and straightforward. You smile ever so slightly, just enough to lift the outside edges of your lips up. If you like, you can think of something mildly funny or someone or something that makes you feel happy. The simple behavior of smiling ever so slightly is enough to activate quiet mind.

As you slip into a half-knowing smile, reflect on the idea that life is tricky, slippery, and actually amusing in its own way. The stresses you're facing in life right now need not be taken so seriously. If you can be playful with them, you might discover new ways of relating to them that give you more emotional freedom and peace of mind. Try the half-knowing smile right now, and practice it as often as you can. It's especially helpful in moments when you're taking stress so seriously that it's getting the better of you. In such circumstances, the half-knowing smile is a nonverbal cue to step back from the situation, look at it from eagle perspective, and love yourself!

Practice: Wrapping Yourself in a Blue Blanket

This practice involves using your imagination. As a warm-up, try imagining a red apple. Are you able to picture the apple? Can you smell it? Perhaps you can even taste your imagined apple. If you're skilled at this type of imagining, this exercise may be a great way to practice loving yourself.

To practice, first imagine that you're in a safe place, about to sit down and rest for a moment. You notice that there's a soft, blue blanket in the chair where you plan to rest. You pick the blanket up and wrap it around you. It's large and covers all of you. It's very smooth, has silky edges, and smells quite nice. Sit down and enjoy being wrapped in the blanket. Let the experience of loving yourself surround and flow over you. Consider practicing this exercise with a real blanket at times so that you can enjoy a direct experience of protection and comfort.

Practice: Feeling Love

Can you remember a time in your life when you felt totally loved and cared for? Can you remember what it felt like to bask in the warmth of being accepted for who you were and being completely connected with your surroundings? In this exercise, we want you to recall these kinds of experiences, then immerse yourself in the memories, including all of the details about the various emotions, thoughts, memories, or physical sensations that this experience created in you. Some people remember being held or gently touched by a parent when they were small. Others remember moments with a partner, such as holding hands and watching a beautiful sunset. Perhaps you have a memory of being hugged by someone who was very glad to see you after a long time apart. Your favorite memories might also involve snuggling with sweet canine or feline friends.

To begin, make a list of moments when you felt really loved, then choose one or two to use in your first practice period. The practice is to remember these events in detail and spend a few moments re-creating the physical, emotional, and mental experience of receiving love. Afterward, describe all of the details of that experience in your journal. Then you can call on those sensations later to deliver that same kind of love to yourself anytime, perhaps especially when you're feeling stressed or self-critical. The experience of loving yourself may be difficult to describe; it may lie more in the realm of sensation and perhaps color. However you experience it, it is love, and it is good brain training.

Practice: Breathing In What You Resist

Practicing self-compassion requires that you see your plight as being the same as the plight of others. It's hard to love yourself if you feel that you are somehow isolated from humanity and on the outside looking in. This exercise, which takes just ten minutes, will guide you in engaging in two distinct forms of compassion. Find a quiet place to practice where you won't be disturbed.

Take a few deep, slow breaths to center yourself. Then, on a very slow inhalation (four to five seconds in duration), hold something that you don't like about yourself in your attention. This might be a traumatic memory, an emotion you find difficult to accept, or a self-critical thought that keeps coming back into your mind. The goal is to voluntarily let go of your resistance to this experience or aspect of yourself. Just let it wash over you and suffuse you without struggling with it.

Next, on a very slow exhalation (again, four to five seconds), turn your attention outward and connect with the suffering of everyone else in the world who's struggling with the same experience that you took in as you inhaled. Try to experience their suffering as you've experienced your own suffering. Can you see your plight as being intimately connected with the plight of others like you? Take a moment to imagine that you aren't alone in your suffering and that there's a bond between you and everyone else facing the same difficulty. There is enormous power in this shared bond. See if you can experience it.

Exercise: You Are Awesome!

People often think that focusing on their good qualities is somehow egotistical and self-centered. Nothing could be further from the truth! The unfortunate reality is that most of restless mind's chatter is negative and self-critical. Therefore, if you don't practice creating positive self-assessments, your mind's circuits will continue to scan for the negative. It's important to offset the natural tendency of restless mind to find faults with you by consciously practicing making contact with the things you love about yourself. To help you with this, we'll ask you to identify your strengths and be grateful for them.

Spend some time listing your strengths and describing why you love them. You'll find a downloadable worksheet for this purpose online at http://www.newharbinger.com/31274 (see the back of this book for instructions on how to access it). Alternatively, you can create a similar form, perhaps in your journal for this book, using the two columns in the downloadable worksheet: "My strength" on the left, and "Why I love it" on the right. If you have difficulty coming up with strengths, picture yourself in situations where your strengths have helped you. You might also picture yourself in situations where one of your strengths (such as caring for others) was a bit of a liability. Accept all of those pictures and, in your mind, express your gratitude to yourself for being a person with strengths and for doing what you do with them.

After completing this portion of the exercise, set aside five to ten minutes to generate positive self-statements based on your strengths, maybe when you wake up in the morning or before you go to bed. At that time, read each strength either aloud or slightly under your breath, pause for a moment, and then say, "I love this about myself!" If restless mind shows up and tries to interfere in any way, such as telling you that you aren't as good as you think you are, thank it for communicating with you and then return to the practice.

Exercise: You Are Flawsome!

In this exercise, you'll practice self-compassion for your personal flaws, both real and imagined. There are two basic types of flaws people tend to beat themselves up about. The first is some attribute that you find unacceptable, be it a receding hairline, stuttering when under stress, or feeling that you aren't as interesting as other people. The second type is something you believe you lack, like good looks, confidence in social situations, or public speaking ability.

Take a few minutes now to identify the flaws you most dislike about yourself, from both categories. For each, try to clearly describe the flaw and what you don't like about it. You'll find a downloadable worksheet for this purpose online at http://www.newharbinger.com/31274. Alternatively, you can create a similar form, perhaps in your journal for this book, using the two columns in the downloadable worksheet: "My flaw" on the left, and "Why it bothers me" on the right.

Once you've identified your flaws, it's time to practice being flawsome! Read each of your flaws out loud, and at the end of each statement, say, "And I love this part of me too!" As you do this, really put yourself into it. See if you can genuinely extend loving energy toward whatever you dislike about yourself. If restless mind tells you that your flaw can't be accepted, practice detachment and gently redirect your attention back to loving yourself. You could even take what restless mind told you, write *that* down as a flaw, and make that part of your flawsomeness! During this practice, try to create a mental space in which you relax, let go of attachment to perfectionism and self-rejection, and truly love what you dislike about yourself.

Practice: Taking Love Breaks

There's a simple principle we want to encourage you to live by during your journey to transcending daily stress: when done consciously, sharing love with others shines a light that also enriches you. We once heard a saying that reflects this basic feedback loop in life: "If you see the face of God in everyone, they will see the face of God in you." Now that you've practiced loving your positive qualities and personal flaws with the same amount of passion, you're in an excellent position to extend this positive energy to the people who are important in your life. However, in the stress-filled, rapid-fire pace of daily life, this may not happen unless you deliberately choose to do so.

There are several ways to pursue the practice of extending love and compassion to those you care about. If you meditate on a daily basis, you can try starting or ending your meditation with a practice of sending love to someone. You can send them "good vibrations" or just think of what you might say or do if you were with that person. Another approach is to write out a daily loving activity plan, each day choosing who your focus will be and what your loving action will be, then writing it down and committing to it.

Whatever form this practice takes for you, it's important to be free of any expectations of reciprocity. Rather, extend love and compassion to others just because you can and you choose to. Loving others in this way helps you train your brain to love yourself, and even to love people who sometimes seem difficult to love. This practice is also immensely helpful when applied to a friend or loved one you're worried about. Replace the fretting with loving!

Practice: Expressing Gratitude

One way to experience self-compassion is to practice being grateful and thankful for even the small things you have in life. When you make a point of doing this on a regular basis, you'll probably be amazed to discover that you actually have a lot of things to be thankful for, even if your mind is working overtime to point out all the things that are going wrong. If you open your mind to it, there are almost unlimited opportunities to experience and express gratitude. Here are a few that we particularly like.

One in the Beginning and One in the End

One of our favorite gratitude practices is something we call "one in the beginning and one in the end." For this practice, upon awakening, express gratitude for whatever enters your awareness. If you hear a dog barking, your beginning might be "I am thankful for dogs." Alternatively, you might not notice the barking dog and instead become aware of the feeling in your eyes—that they are rested and ready to begin the day: "I am thankful for my eyes." The morning practice is "one in the beginning." "One in the end" refers to doing the same practice when you lie down at night to go to sleep. If you're aware of your soft, favorite pillow, you could express gratitude by softly saying, "I am thankful for my pillow."

While you may benefit from simply thinking these thoughts of gratitude, consider experimenting with saying them aloud or writing them in your journal—or even keeping a special gratitude journal.

Daily Review

Another type of gratitude practice is the daily review. Before you go to bed at night, practice a two- to three-minute reflection on what you were thankful for that day. Try to think of things that happened that enriched you as a human being, even if ever so slightly. Maybe someone held a door open for you or greeted you with a smile. Maybe something stressful happened and you used the situation to practice a new skill. Practicing gratitude for the little things in daily life creates grace and the eagle perspective that we encourage you to cultivate.

Gratitude for Your Past

A third option is to back up a bit and express gratitude toward a teacher or another important person in your past whose influence is still with you today. Alternatively, you can cultivate gratitude for past situations, even those that caused a lot of personal pain but also taught you a lot about yourself. Can you express gratitude toward this type of circumstance in your life? It's worth giving it a go. After all, the alternative is to carry around a negative, judgmental narrative about how you were hurt or damaged. How does the emotion tone of that story compare with a stance of experiencing gratitude for the opportunity to learn more about who you are, for better or for worse? Just check it out!

Exercise: Seeing Your Life as a Novel

Learning to relate to your personal narrative from eagle perspective is a critical component of loving yourself. As your life unfolds, your personal narrative functions as a kind of life novel that's being written second by second. The key thing about writing (or reading) a novel is character development. As readers, we delight in watching the hero or heroine grow in strength and stature through life experiences, even painful ones. If you treat your life like it's a novel unfolding in front of you, it creates a sense of continuity between what was, what is, and what will be. As it turns out, you, and only you, are the author of this novel!

For this exercise, you'll step back and look at the different eras of your life as though they were, are, or will be chapters in your life novel. Take some time to reflect on your life, keeping in mind that this is your novel and you can love every chapter of it, even those that are painful and perplexing. After reflecting on your life, answer the questions below, which will guide you in describing your life novel. Some of the questions ask you to assign titles; for these, keep your responses simple yet descriptive.

- *What's the title of your life novel?*

- *What are the titles of the chapters that have been written so far, from earliest to most recent?*

- *What's the title of the chapter you're currently living?*

- *What are the major life themes (section headings) for the current chapter, and what is the hero or heroine learning about life and himself or herself?*

- *What's your least favorite chapter so far?*

- *Is there a way for you to feel more love for the person you were in your least favorite chapter?*

- *What are the titles for the chapters you'll write in the remainder of your life novel?*

Practice Makes Permanent

In this section, we'll help you write out your commitment to practicing the exercises in this chapter. Practicing self-compassion on a regular basis will help you to live your day-to-day life with more self-acceptance and less self-criticism. You'll discover that the practice of loving yourself opens new doors for you in all arenas of your life. Let's face it: walking around feeling good about who you are (and aren't) is much better than rejecting yourself. Plus, when you can love yourself, it will be much easier to extend compassion to others and make room for their shortcomings. It's well worth devoting some time and effort to training your mind to walk the path of self-compassion. Take a moment to plan your practice by considering the following questions and writing your responses in your journal:

- What brain training practices or exercises do you plan to use?

- When will you practice? Be specific: note the date and time of day for planned practices.

- Who will be your ally in practice, and what type of support will you request?

- How will you celebrate your first week of practice?

Gentle Reminders

Learning to love yourself, or practicing self-compassion, is a high-level mindfulness skill that is a key aspect of any approach to transcending daily stress. Part of the stress of being human is that you aren't perfect; you can and will make mistakes or disappoint yourself or others. Self-compassion involves accepting the fact that you have flaws, make mistakes, and aren't perfect, while still treating yourself with love and kindness. Doing so requires you to detach from and be curious about the harsh, critical self-narratives of restless mind and its tendency to remind you of your faults. When you practice self-compassion instead, you strengthen the neural circuitry that allows you to enter into a state of quiet mind, with love and self-acceptance washing over you.

In the end, the choice to love or hate yourself is completely up to you, and you can choose to switch from self-loathing to loving yourself at any time, and for no reason at all! If you do so, you'll be in a good position to create a deliberate and self-accepting approach to acting mindfully in daily life. This is another important skill to acquire as part of your program for transcending daily stress, and the topic of the next chapter, so read on!

CHAPTER 8

Act Mindfully

If you take care of the minutes, the years will take care of themselves.

—Buddhist saying

In this chapter, you'll learn skills for living deliberately, in the progression of moments of your daily life, and in a way that's consistent with your beliefs and principles for living. Ultimately, this is the most important step you can take to transcend daily stress: making an ongoing commitment to living life on purpose, based upon what's important to you, rather than in reaction to the stress you're under. This puts stress in its proper perspective in the bigger picture of your life. Most of the stresses you're facing today won't be here a year from now, and in hindsight, you might see your struggles in a completely different light than you do today.

As you embark on this journey, one challenge you'll face is that living with everyday stress may make you shortsighted. People tend to adapt to stress by letting go of important life goals or forgetting them and instead just trying to make it from one day to the next. This style of living can leave you preoccupied with stress-related negative emotions, unpleasant physical symptoms, and self-critical thinking. In this scenario, stress is essentially dictating the terms and conditions of how you experience life.

Although living day to day might be a convenient way of coping with daily stress and all of the related problems you might be facing, your nervous system isn't designed to live this way over the long haul. Plus, most of us don't do well when we have no sense of a bigger purpose in life than making it to the next paycheck or trying to get through another week of housework and parenting. This can sap your motivation to get out and smell the roses. We all need to show up in our lives and base our lifestyles in the principles we want to live by.

Your mission, should you choose to accept it, is to begin living life deliberately, on purpose, and in the moment. In this chapter, we'll help you create a different vision of daily living, one that can encompass stress and still allow you to experience a sense of vitality, purpose, and meaning in life.

Core Components of Acting Mindfully

Acting mindfully involves two core processes, and they will be the focus of the exercises and practices in this chapter. First, acting mindfully requires that you slow down, show up, and become aware of a specific purpose that you will embody in your behavior in the moment. This purpose can be as simple as choosing to savor the taste of each bite of an apple as you eat it slowly, or as difficult as consciously choosing to speak and act compassionately as you confront your next-door neighbors about an issue involving their teenage son.

Second, acting mindfully requires that you persist with behaviors that are linked to your specific purpose, even when obstacles show up. To use a popular term in the culture of everyday stress, you must be able to multitask—and do so without losing sight of what you intend to do and care about doing. There's a well-worn saying that sums up this ironic feature of life: "Life is what happens to us while we are making other plans" (Saunders 1957, 32).

Ultimately, the real value of living in the moment is what you learn about yourself when you try to do so. You're likely to discover that living in the moment is where vitality and meaning lie, rather than in how much money you make, how popular or attractive you are, how lavish or adventurous your vacations are, or how high up the corporate ladder you climb.

The Perspective of Intention

Acting mindfully requires that you act with intention, which in turn requires that you focus your attention on a specific goal and then organize your actions to move in the direction of that goal. People often think of goals as existing in the future, but in reality some of the most powerful types of intentional action happen immediately, in the moment. Consider athletic achievement: World-class athletes often describe themselves as being "in the zone" during a peak, record-setting performance. In the zone, the pace of mental processing doesn't speed up; it slows down. Information seems to be coming into the mind at a slower, more measured pace even though, in reality, nothing has changed in the outside word. We are dialed in, as the saying goes. Attention and intention are perfectly balanced.

One of the aspects of acting mindfully that's difficult to grasp is that when you deliberately slow down, focus, and act with intention, you aren't falling behind. You're actually pulling ahead. In the end, it isn't about how fast things are moving; it's about mental efficiency. When you practice intentional action, you make contact with the challenges of daily stress in a highly organized and efficient way. You process information much more accurately, you're less distracted by irrelevant information, and your behavior is more precise and purposeful.

Thus, acting mindfully has a flexible, fluid quality that allows you to respond in a highly organized, effective way when you're under stress. Doing so calls upon all of the mindfulness skills we explored in chapters 4 through 7. When you need to observe, you observe. When you need to describe, you describe. When detachment is needed, you detach. When self-compassion is called for, you practice self-compassion. And when it comes time to act, you act. Make this your new mantra for transcending daily stress: Pay attention and act with intention!

The Neuropsychology of Intention

The ability to create intentional, goal-directed behavior is a cognitive activity: linking a mentally constructed goal to organized, ongoing patterns of behavior. It originates in highly complex synchronous neural circuitry located in both the lateral prefrontal cortex and the lateral occipital complex—areas of the brain that are critical to effective problem solving during times of stress, when there are usually many potential barriers to effective action. Activation of these areas supports semantic memory processing (converting abstract life principles into specific behavioral goals), processing of cause and effect relations (determining whether a specific action is likely to achieve the imagined goal), and motivational processing (evaluating the feasibility of taking the imagined action).

It appears that the activities of mental rehearsal and subsequent organization of behavior are very closely connected. Therefore, we encourage you to mentally rehearse important goal-oriented behaviors prior to engaging in them. Interestingly, the number and complexity of neural connections in the areas of the brain supporting purposeful behavior increase with age, suggesting that we become progressively more capable of acting with intention as a result of the brain training that life gives us. Not a bad payoff for all the indignities we have to endure as we age!

A concept that is currently in vogue in cognitive neuroscience is *working memory capacity*, which refers to the ability to stay focused on a task even while irrelevant or distracting information is coming in from other sectors of your awareness. For example, you can receive and respond to a text from a friend or family member while participating in a project meeting at work. You can shift your attention rapidly between the text message and the content of the work meeting without losing the ability to participate effectively in either task. Working memory capacity is particularly important in addressing the multiple and often competing demands of daily stress. The higher your working memory capacity is, the more easily you can shift your attention back and forth while focusing your energy and behavior on what matters in the moment.

The Neuroscience of Acting Mindfully

The core skills involved in acting mindfully, the underlying neural circuits, and the associated mental processes are outlined below.

Mindful action skill: Taking actions consistent with an immediate self-experienced purpose

Areas of the brain involved

- Lateral orbitofrontal cortex

- Medial orbitofrontal cortex

- Anterior cingulate nucleus

Mental processes

- Linking mental representations of actions with correlated motor movements

- Constructing and evaluating the positive and negative consequences of mentally represented actions

Mindful action skill: Persisting with intentional actions despite distracting input

Areas of the brain involved

- Superior frontal sulcus

- Posterior parietal cortex

- Posterior cingulate cortex/precuneus

Mental processes

- Maintaining goal-directed behavior when faced with task distractions

- Allowing for selective shifting of attention and processing resources based on task demands

Brain Training

When you practice acting mindfully, you activate neural circuits that operate in reciprocal feedback loops. Whatever goes through these loops is strengthened and amplified in the underlying neural circuitry. A long line of research has shown that the more you practice a behavior, the easier it is to do it again. The neural basis for forming new habits resides in the brain's ability to functionally link neurons that are repeatedly involved in performing the same activity. There's a saying in neuroscientific circles, attributed to Carla Shatz, a highly respected neuroscientist, that makes this point better than we can: "Neurons that fire together, wire together" (Doidge 2007, 63).

The brain training exercises we provide in this chapter will help you fire neurons that govern intention, choice, and mindful action together—and in a variety of different ways. As you practice these exercises, you'll find it increasingly easy to behave mindfully and intentionally in more and more areas of your life.

Practice: Deliberance

Deliberance is a funky derivative of the word "deliverance" that a stressed-out client once used to describe his daily habit of singling out seemingly mundane tasks and doing them mindfully and on purpose. In this exercise, you'll mindfully engage in routines that you usually don't pay much attention to. Targets for deliberance training include routine daily tasks like eating meals, washing dishes, fixing stuff around the house, and so forth. Doing things deliberately requires that you show up, get into the moment, and then pay attention to what you're doing as you do it.

Listed below are some areas in your daily routine where you might apply the deliberance fix:

- *Getting out of bed in the morning*

- *Eating meals*

- *Taking walks*

- *Washing dishes*

- *Doing laundry*

- *Eating lunch at work*

- *Tending to houseplants*

- *Working in your yard*

- *Sweeping the floor*

- *Doing household repairs*

- *Engaging in your bedtime routine*

Choose one or two routine daily tasks to focus on, whether from the list or otherwise. Then make a plan for how you'll do these tasks more intentionally. To strengthen your commitment, be sure to write your plans down, either in your journal or on the downloadable worksheet for this exercise—which you can find online at http://www.newhar binger.com/31274 (see the back of this book for instructions on how to access it).

Practice: Taking Twice as Long

When you're stressed-out, it's likely that you'll do many of your daily activities automatically and without much awareness, just racing to get things done. In this mind-set, how you do tasks is typically much less important than completing them. This exercise will help you vary this pattern by deliberately changing your pace—actually going for taking twice as long as usual.

Pick any of the routine daily activities listed in the previous exercise, Deliberance, and try to do it at about half speed, so that it takes you twice as long. The intention in slowing down is to make conscious contact with each action you engage in while completing the task. If you choose eating a meal as your target, you'd focus on every behavior you engage in to eat: reaching, lifting, opening your mouth, chewing, tasting, and so on. See if you can get into a zone where you're aware of and study each action, almost like you're becoming aware of the action for the first time.

This is quite likely to trigger restless mind, so you might hear messages to hurry up and get this task finished because you don't have time to dally! If you notice this happening, detach from that message and see it as just a message. You can always speed up again in a few minutes, after completing this task. However, you might notice that it's actually kind of fun, not to mention good for your mental health, to slow down and get into the mindful action zone.

Exercise: Identifying What Matters

By now, it should be clear that living with daily stress can result in living life small—just coping with each day, one day at a time. Yet this strategy feeds stress, because it's stressful to feel like your life is constricted and lacks space for play, self-exploration, and growth. We want to help you expand the scope of your life so it's rich in opportunities for self-growth. The first step in acting with intention is to figure out what really matters to you in life.

To do this exercise (based on Hayes, Strosahl, and Wilson 1999, and Strosahl and Robinson 2008), consider the areas listed below, then write down any important life goals in these areas, either in your journal or on the downloadable worksheet for this exercise, which you can find online at http://www.newharbinger.com/31274. Note that this isn't a timed test; the goal isn't to get to the end of the exercise as fast as you can. Do it thoughtfully and mindfully, taking the time you need.

- *Work, study, and career pursuits*

- *Intimate relationships*

- *Family relationships*

- *Friendships*

- *Relaxation and leisure pursuits*

- *Spiritual development*

- *Contribution to social good*

- *Personal growth and development*

- *Health and well-being*

We recommend repeating this exercise on a regular basis, perhaps doing it as part of some occasion that's important to you, like your wedding anniversary, your birthday, or a religious holiday. This will help you to stay in tune with what matters to you as well as to stick with your goals as they change through time. Remember, the road to acting mindfully starts by forming mental images of how your life could be if you keep pursuing what matters to you.

Practice: Stating Your Intentions Out Loud

Instead of just trying to survive another day in the stress zone, with this practice you'll choose something that matters to you in your life to connect your intention to. At the beginning of your day, pause for a few minutes and try to visualize opportunities for slowing down, showing up, and engaging in some type of behavior that reflects what's important to you in your life. Then express your intentions out loud and make a commitment to follow through with them. For example, say you intend to talk with your partner about something that made you laugh, doing so as part of a bigger life goal of promoting intimacy in your relationship. In that case, you'd say to yourself, out loud, "Today, I'm going to talk with my partner about something that made me laugh. I'm doing this because I want to create a more loving relationship."

Practice: Enjoying Yourself

Stress tends to rob us of our ability to simply enjoy daily life and the activities that go into it. This exercise involves choosing a context in your life where you want to be more playful so that you can enjoy yourself even when stress is present. For example, you might choose work. Then consider a variety of activities that are playful that you could plan to do at work, such as telling a joke (even if you read it from a piece of paper) or doing a little dance when you enter the break room. If, as you engage in this act, your mind tells you it's a waste of time to be spontaneous and silly, thank your mind and immediately engage in another behavior that has no redeeming value beyond play. We need to warn you that this exercise may have an impact on people around you. Your lightheartedness and obvious enjoyment of just being alive may provoke playful responding in others. Alternatively, some people may try to get you to snap out of it and be oh-so-serious again. If this happens, you can enjoy putting on that oh-so-serious face again and showing everyone how oh-so-serious you can be!

Exercise: Creating a Vision-Action Plan

As discussed earlier, the neural circuitry of intention seems to combine the activities of imagined life outcomes and real behavior in one seamless process. This suggests that the natural way to train your brain to act mindfully is first to create a vision of the future, whether one minute from now or forty years from now, and then create a mental action plan that would help you achieve that vision. If you create a very specific action plan and make a commitment to follow it, you're likely to succeed even if unexpected barriers arise.

To do this exercise, start by reviewing your responses to the previous exercise and contemplating what matters to you. Then take it a step further and, for each area, identify a specific action you'll take to bring your life into greater alignment with what matters to you. To strengthen your commitment, be sure to write your plans down, either in your journal or on the downloadable worksheet for this exercise, which you can find online at http://www.newharbinger.com/31274. Be as specific as possible when describing these actions, stating when you intend to do them, how often you'll do them, and so forth.

Exercise: Checking Your Compass Heading

One of the sneakiest impacts of stress is that it can slowly take you off track in terms of what matters to you, and you may not notice that this is happening until you're way off course. Of course, this adds to your stress because, at some level, you experience the dissonance. This exercise will help you monitor the direction of your life journey on an ongoing basis so you can make course corrections easily when daily stresses tend take you off on tangents.

For the purposes of this exercise, let's call the life direction you want to be heading toward true north. When you're headed toward your own, personal true north, you're living in a way that's completely consistent with the things in life that matter most to you. You can use the results of the two preceding exercises to help you develop your definition of true north. This might involve combining your aspirations in several life areas into one bigger statement about how you want to live your life.

On a fresh page in your journal or a separate piece of paper (or using the downloadable True North Worksheet available at http://www.newharbinger.com/31274), write your statement about your true north near the top of the page, then draw a box around the statement to enclose it. Underneath the box, draw a big circle with the basic compass headings: north at the top, pointing directly to the box with your true north statement; east 90 degrees to the right; south at the bottom, directly opposite north; and west on the left, midway between south and north. We'll call this your life compass.

The direction you want to be headed in is true north, but if you're like most people (us included!), you're at least a little bit off course. Place a mark on your compass to designate the direction you think you're traveling right now. If you see that you're off course, please remember to bring self-compassion to this exercise. Also, realize that while some parts of you may be off course, other parts are undoubtedly headed straight toward true north.

Now take a moment to write about the strategies you're currently using to move in the direction of your values and whether they're working. If your current course is heading significantly away from true north, also write about mental or real-world obstacles that may be causing you to get off course.

Now consider this: What would it take for you to move yourself, even if just a bit at a time, in the direction of true north, with those obstacles present? Come up with a specific action plan for correcting your course, then write it down. While something like "I could spend more time with my children even though I'm stressed-out after work" is a good start, it isn't specific enough to ensure success. So get detailed;

for example, "I intend to spend at least thirty minutes with my children after work each weekday, regardless of whether I'm tired or not." The more specific your course-correction plan is, the more deliberately and purposefully you'll be in acting on it.

Once you've developed a specific plan, state your intention out loud. Also consider enlisting the support of a friend or family member or your partner to keep you accountable. We recommend repeating this exercise regularly. After all, no one makes the journey through life without veering off course fairly often.

Practice: Revamping Your Lifestyle

Just as the effects of daily stress can quickly compound and take a huge toll on health and well-being, so too can the effects of daily lifestyle choices. The good news here is that although you often can't control stressors, you can control daily decisions about diet, exercise, relaxation, sleep, and taking time for yourself.

What you eat can either heighten or relieve stress, so consider your eating habits. If you tend to go for fast food at the last minute because you're always running late, this is a gigantic message that you aren't in control of your life. Study up on what you need to eat to live vitally. Take a cooking class or join a circle supper group for support in preparing more healthful food and eating more intentionally.

Likewise, physical activity, or lack thereof, can have a huge impact not only on how you cope with daily stress but also on your physical and mental well-being. We know that regular exercise improves cardiovascular health, makes people less susceptible to everyday illnesses, helps control weight, and produces a positive state of mind. Exercise releases neuropeptides called endorphins, which are one of the brain's natural opioids. Public health experts regard regular exercise as the single most important health protective behavior you can engage in.

Also consider issues like the quality of your water, the air you breathe, the lighting in your home or at work, and so on. People often think things like this are beyond their control, but if you want to do something to improve your immediate environment, you can.

Take some time to consider your options for making any long overdue changes to your lifestyle both at home and at work. In your journal, list the possibilities, then identify a few lifestyle changes to start working on. You might want to begin with small, easily achievable steps, such as getting a water filter. Or you may want to target actions in areas that hold the potential for major positive changes, such as exercising on a regular basis. Whatever you choose, consider working with friends, family members, or others who might join you in taking action to improve your lifestyle.

Practice Makes Permanent

In this section, we'll help you write out your commitment to practicing the exercises in this chapter. Approaching your daily activities with intention and mindfulness will help you live your day-to-day life with more joy and peace of mind, and more resilience against daily stress. You can train your nervous system to strengthen the neural connections that link vision and action, allowing your mind to create more powerful, life-affirming visions of the future. Your brain can work for you, not against you, in everyday life, day in, day out. Take a moment to plan your practice by considering the following questions and writing your responses in your journal:

- What brain training practices or exercises do you plan to use?

- When will you practice? Be specific: Note the date and time of day.

- Who will be your ally in practice, and what type of support will you request?

- How will you celebrate your first week of practice?

Gentle Reminders

Learning to act mindfully and with intention is a powerful step toward living a life that matters to you. Acting mindfully means doing things more deliberately, and this requires ongoing brain training. A strong connection with your personal principles and beliefs can give you direction when stress runs high. Remember to slow down and do what matters when addressing daily hassles. You can engage in mindful action in any moment, and even with routine household activities, such as washing dishes, caring for plants in your house or yard, or feeding your pet.

Mindful action also involves creating a long-term vision of the life you'd like to be living and developing daily routines that help you live in a way that's consistent with that vision. The beauty of acting mindfully is that it can be used to organize both short-term and long-term approaches to living a fulfilling, vital life. In part 3 of this book, we'll help you engage in a series of lifestyle changes that will increase your ability to transcend stress and also have long-lasting benefits for you and those you care about.

PART 3

Developing a Mindful Lifestyle

CHAPTER 9

Know Your Helpers and Hassles

Don't visualize success. Instead, visualize the
steps you will take in order to succeed.

—Heidi Grant Halvorson

In the final chapters of this book, we'll help you put together a specific, sustainable lifestyle plan that will help you transcend daily stress and live a more vital, meaningful life. We'll guide you through a straightforward sequence of tasks, devoting a short chapter to each step. First, you need to take an inventory of the daily stressors, or hassles, you're currently experiencing, as well as the strategies you employ to offset stress—your daily helpers. Second, we'll help you use this information to create a more mindful lifestyle that provides you with the self-care and self-restoration you need to transcend stress. Third, we'll guide you in developing a system for applying your mindfulness skills to work or school endeavors, as well as to your efforts to give something back to your community. Finally, we'll help you figure out how to moderate the effects of daily stress on your relationships and instead create a mindful tone in your interactions with others.

If you approach these four chapters with intention and patience, collectively they will help you implement a complete lifestyle transformation. When you combine this with the brain training exercises in part 2 of this book, you'll have a very powerful one-two punch in your battle to transcend daily stress!

For several decades, stress experts have argued that the impact of daily hassles is reduced in direct proportion to a person's ability to engage in daily helpers (Kanner et al. 1981; Holm and Holroyd 1992).

To a large degree, your overall level of stress is determined by your ratio of hassles to helpers. You can almost think of this as your overall stress index.

In this chapter, we'll start with the important initial task of helping you assess your ratio of helpers to hassles and share some practical ideas about what to do to make this ratio more favorable. We'll have you complete three fairly in-depth self-assessments, and the results of these assessments will inform your work in the final three chapters of the book.

The first assessment involves identifying the helpers and hassles within your current lifestyle. The second assessment asks you to evaluate the relative power or impact of helpers and hassles in core areas of your day-to-day life. The final assessment looks at how much control you have over individual helpers or hassles and will help you consider two different ways of responding based upon this dimension. For those helpers and hassles over which you have limited or no control, you generally need to practice acceptance so you don't waste valuable time and energy pushing against the river, so to speak. For those over which you have a great deal of control, you can systematically build new habits to establish a new lifestyle. To intentionally change the way you respond to stress or enhance your state of mind, it's best to embed new behaviors in the basic contexts of life: self-care, work, and relationships. The final three chapters of the book will help you do just that.

To begin, pull together the information you've already generated in earlier exercises: the data you've collected in your Daily Hassles and Helpers Log and the action plans you generated at the end of each of the chapters in part 2 of this book. This information will be invaluable for identifying possible helpers and hassles that either support or challenge your ability to choose a mindful response instead of letting stress dictate your lifestyle.

Daily Helpers

Daily helpers are activities that stimulate quiet mind and therefore help reduce emotional and physiological arousal and create greater peace of mind. Helpers can take many forms and may involve mental, physical, or social activities. Many of the mindfulness skills introduced in part 2 of this book are mental helpers. They typically slow down automatic responses and promote more relaxed and flexible behavior, which not only feels better but also often promotes relaxed and flexible behavior in others. In addition, you may already engage in mental practices that are helpful, such as prayer or inspirational reading, alone or with others. These are valuable daily helpers, so keep them in your tool kit!

You may also have physical daily helpers, such as going for a morning walk or daily jog or taking a yoga class several times a week. Other physical daily helpers include tai chi, tae kwan do, weight training, and aerobics classes. Physical helpers provide many benefits, so if you're light on these, consider beefing up in this area. One suggestion regarding physical helpers is that you do them mindfully. For example, you might choose to focus on your breath throughout a yoga class or a swim. Another approach is to set an intention for a physical activity (for example, "My intention in this run is to touch the earth lightly") or to participate in activities associated with benefits to others (such as running or walking for a cause).

Interactions with others can also pack a powerful punch in helping you to transcend stress. Examples include attending group meetings (with others who share common values) or participating in volunteer activities. An especially helpful approach is to have a partner to support you in making the lifestyle changes you decide upon. If you take this approach, don't hesitate to be specific about the kind of support you're looking for. For example, you might say, "Please be available to me for thirty minutes each weekend to just listen while I let off steam about various stresses, particularly those I have no control over. After you listen for five or ten minutes, smile and say something like "I know you can let this go. What's your plan for resetting mentally and physically?"

Exercise: Identifying Daily Helpers

This exercise will help you identify your daily helpers. To jog your memory of helpers that may already be present in your everyday life, take a look at the following lists, which show some common helpers (Kanner et al. 1981). We've divided them into two basic categories: those with a personal focus and those with a social or work focus.

Consider whether each is making a positive contribution to your life, and check off any that are.

Personal focus

_____ Laughing

_____ Enjoying entertainment (e.g., movies, the theater, concerts)

_____ Painting or doing other artwork or crafts

_____ Celebrating your physical appearance, such as having fun with dressing

_____ Playing or listening to music

_____ Journaling

_____ Meditating

_____ Doing yoga

_____ Doing breathing practices

_____ Going to church

_____ Taking time for yourself

_____ Doing an enjoyable hobby

_____ Exercising

_____ Taking a slow walk and enjoying the sights

_____ Taking care of plants

_____ Eating healthy food

_____ Getting enough sleep

_____ Reading a good book

Social or work focus

_____ Relating well with your partner

_____ Relating well with friends

_____ Completing a difficult task at work

_____ Getting a compliment from your boss or supervisor

_____ Getting a compliment from your partner

_____ Shopping with someone

_____ Eating with your partner or family

_____ Meeting responsibilities at home

_____ Playing games with friends or family

_____ Visiting, calling, or texting someone

_____ Dancing or roughhousing with someone

_____ Doing a fun project at home with family members

_____ Watching a comedy show or TV series with someone

_____ Getting or giving love or cuddling

_____ Being visited, phoned, or texted by a friend

_____ Playing or interacting with a pet

Now take a few moments to think about other daily helpers in your life. If you've been keeping a Daily Hassles and Helpers Log, that information will be useful here. For this exercise, we'll ask you to list your daily helpers, then categorize them and rate their impact. You'll find a downloadable worksheet for this purpose at http://www.newharbinger. com/31274 (see the back of the book for instructions on how to access it). Alternatively, you can create a similar form, perhaps in your journal for this book, using the four columns in the downloadable worksheet: "Day of week and time" on the left, then "Daily helper," then "Category (personal, social, work)," and finally "Helper impact" on the right. For "Helper impact," rate how effective each helper is using a scale of 1 to 5, where 1 is just a bit helpful and 5 is very helpful.

The Challenge: Living with Daily Hassles

As mentioned in part 1 of this book, there's growing evidence that the accumulation of daily hassles, those annoying everyday stresses we must live with, has a bigger effect on mental and physical well-being than major life events such as divorce or job loss. We think the reason for this counterintuitive finding lies in the term "daily." Because these are daily events, and because they seem to be (or really are) beyond our control, we learn to ignore them or avoid dealing with our emotional responses to them, often at a real cost to mental and physical health.

For the purposes of your work in this chapter, think of daily hassles as fitting into four broad categories: personal concerns, relationship and family concerns, work or school concerns, and social or environmental concerns. Those categories are fairly self-descriptive, but here's a bit more information about each, in case you find it helpful. Personal concerns include a multitude of self-oriented things you might struggle with in daily life, ranging from uncertainty about your direction in life to worries about your health or finances. Relationship and family hassles include daily stresses that arise from your role or interactions in various relationships, such as with your partner, children, other family members, and close friends. Work and school concerns range from conflicts you might be having with coworkers to the feeling that you might need to drop an important required course at school because you don't have enough time to complete the homework. Social and environmental concerns can range from local to global in scale, such as dealing with noise pollution in your neighborhood or concerns about water quality to concerns about social injustice and war.

Exercise: Identifying Daily Hassles

For this exercise, we want you to apply your newly developed mindfulness skills to the task of paying attention to all of the daily events that raise your blood pressure or throw you off balance, including seemingly minor stressors. What gets under your skin, and when? Below, we've listed some common daily hassles in the four categories outlined above (Kanner et al. 1981). Read through them, consider whether each is encroaching on your life, and check off any that are.

Personal concerns

_____ *Experiencing inner conflicts*

_____ *Regretting past decisions*

_____ *Feeling conflicted about what to do in life*

_____ *Feeling lonely*

_____ *Feeling unable to express yourself to others*

_____ *Fearing rejection*

_____ *Having trouble making decisions*

_____ *Being concerned about your physical appearance*

_____ *Having a limited social circle*

_____ *Having troubling thoughts about the future*

_____ *Not having enough energy*

_____ *Being concerned about getting ahead*

_____ *Fearing confrontation*

_____ *Wasting time*

_____ *Being concerned about financial credit*

_____ *Not having enough money for food*

_____ *Not having enough money for transportation*

_____ *Having worries about paying bills*

_____ *Not having enough time or money for relaxing and leisure activities*

_____ *Being concerned about owing money*

_____ *Having too many things to do*

_____ *Not having enough time to keep up with responsibilities*

_____ Not getting enough sleep

_____ Being interrupted too often

_____ Not getting enough rest and relaxation

_____ Being concerned about your physical health

_____ Experiencing chronic pain

_____ Dealing with unpleasant medical procedures

_____ Having trouble with taking medications or their side effects

Intimate and family relationships

_____ Having problems with children at home

_____ Children having problems at school

_____ Conflicts with your partner or ex about your children

_____ Keeping up with yard work or home maintenance

_____ Financing your children's education

_____ Being overloaded with family responsibilities

_____ Keeping up with household tasks

_____ Taking care of everyone else's needs

_____ Feeling like you do everything around the house

_____ Not having much intimacy with your partner

_____ Having disagreements about money

_____ Being uncertain about the future of your relationship with your partner

_____ Lacking shared common interests with your partner

_____ Problems with the health or behaviors of pets

_____ Conflicts with your partner or family members about pets

Work or school

_____ *Being hassled by your boss or supervisor*

_____ *Not liking your current work duties*

_____ *Not being able to keep up with course work*

_____ *Not liking coworkers*

_____ *Being unemployed or underemployed*

_____ *Having difficulties juggling study time and family time*

_____ *Not being paid fairly*

_____ *Worrying about whether to change jobs*

_____ *Customers or clients giving you a hard time*

_____ *Having trouble getting along with a coworker*

_____ *Dealing with an annoying classmate*

_____ *Dealing with sexism, ageism, or racism*

_____ *Having problems with employees you supervise*

_____ *Dealing with an uninspired or boring teacher*

_____ *Attending too many meetings at work*

_____ *Peers or employees not getting work done on time*

_____ *Working overtime*

_____ *Spending excessive time commuting to and from work*

Social and environmental concerns

_____ *Concerns about air or pollution and personal health*

_____ *Lacking access to parks and recreational areas*

_____ *Lacking access to health care*

_____ Concerns about crime and personal safety

_____ Dealing with traffic congestion

_____ Concerns about traffic safety

_____ Concerns about recent news events

_____ Dealing with rising costs of basic goods

_____ Concerns about local, state, or national politics

_____ Concerns about climate change and other global environmental problems

_____ Concerns about social injustice

Now take some time to think about any other daily hassles you face. If you've been keeping a Daily Hassles and Helpers Log, that information will be useful here. If you haven't, take a day or two to pay attention to daily hassles as they naturally appear in your life. Some daily hassles are closely tied to duties at work or at home, but they're not confined to these duties, either. They can even show up when you're engaging in leisure activities—organizing everyone in the household, for example, so you can get to a movie on time and not be late. Tracking daily hassles for a few days will help you identify such hassles, and ones that are tied to variations in your routines or those of others you live with or are close to.

For this exercise, we'll ask you to list your daily hassles, categorize them, and rate their impact and the extent to which they're controllable. You'll find a downloadable worksheet for this purpose at http://www.newharbinger.com/31274. Alternatively, you can create a similar form, perhaps in your journal for this book, using the five columns in the downloadable worksheet: "Day of week and time" on the left, then "Daily hassle," then "Category (personal, relationships, work or school, and social or environmental)." The last two columns are "Hassle impact" and, on the far right, "Controllability."

For "Hassle impact," rate how stressful each hassle is using a scale of 1 to 5, where 1 is just a bit stressful and 5 is very stressful. For example, if one of your hassles is excessive household duties, this may have impacts beyond your stress in the moment. It might mean you feel you don't have time for exercise, increasing its overall impact. For "Controllability," indicate how controllable each hassle is by simply stating low, medium, or high. Low indicates that you have little or no control over the hassle, medium indicates that you have some control over whether it occurs, and high means you have a lot of control over it. Taking into account the impact and controllability of any particular hassle is often the first step in forming a plan for making changes and acting more mindfully and effectively.

Pay particular attention to how you describe each hassle. It may be worthwhile to take a few minutes to write freely about your hassles so you can develop more appreciation for their nuances. Be curious! You may unexpectedly notice something that can clue you in to a potentially more effective, stress-transcending response.

A Road Map for Transcending Daily Hassles

In creating a road map for transcending stress, the first principle to consider is that whatever you do in response to daily hassles is part of your action plan, whether you intend it that way or not. Thus, the question isn't whether you're taking steps; it's whether your action plan is working. At times, your reactions may increase rather than decrease the impacts of hassles. For example, if household duties take up so much time that you feel you can't exercise, you might react by becoming short or irritable with your children or partner. In this case, you're responding to one hassle (excessive household duties that get in the way of exercising) by creating another hassle (straining your relationships with family members).

Our hope is that your increasing mindfulness skills will allow you to notice when reactions to stress are creating new hassles, and then perhaps chuckle or at least adopt a half-knowing smile to stimulate your PNS. Although brain training can't create perfection in your daily behavior, it can help you consider other responses that will help you transcend stress in the moment. It may also allow you to anticipate similar stressors in the future so you can cue yourself to respond more mindfully or even rearrange your schedule to prevent the problem. How you choose to respond will often be governed by whether you can control a particular hassle, so let's revisit that issue.

Accept What You Cannot Control

Often there's no easy fix for a particular daily hassle—for example, living in a part of town where you have a very lengthy commute. It could take a long time to either find a job closer to your home or move closer to work. In the meantime, you have to work within yourself to minimize the daily impact of that hassle on your mental and physical well-being.

This is where acceptance is called for. Acceptance is about letting go, and letting go mindfully means letting go with every breath and counting those breaths—honestly! When you find yourself stuck in trying to control something you cannot control, we strongly recommend that you take a moment to breathe mindfully and say "Let go" as you inhale, and "Let grace" as you exhale, with a goal of staying present for ten breaths.

Personally, we've both also found it helpful to post the Serenity Prayer in visible places both at home and at work. If you aren't familiar with it, the Serenity Prayer goes like this: "Grant me the serenity to accept the things I cannot change, the courage to change the things I can, and the wisdom to know the difference." This powerful saying reminds us that there are many things that we cannot control, and that it's best to direct our energy toward responsible action on things we *can* meaningfully influence.

Change What You Can!

Our first principle for coping with daily hassles is that you always have control over your behavior! In the midst of a swarm of daily hassles, you can still create and implement a plan for responding to hassles. Remember, daily stress typically leads to habitual and often counterproductive ways of coping. Therefore, the task at hand is to develop new, more effective habits to combat older ones that don't work well. There are three basic principles involved in acquiring new habits: envisioning the future, thinking small, and accumulating positives.

Envision the Future; Start with the Present

It's easy to get frustrated and impatient with yourself when you're under a lot of pressure due to daily hassles. This might tempt you to take a heroic but unsustainable approach to developing new coping strategies. For example, say you currently don't exercise at all, and you resolve to start exercising five days a week over the next week or two. The odds of being successful with this type of grand change are pretty low. A host of new behaviors are involved in exercising five times a week; and many of them actually have nothing to do with exercising, but rather involve overcoming physical or mental barriers to exercising in the first place. We think it's crucial to have an end goal in mind while also acknowledging that you can only start from where you are, not where you'd like to be. This leads nicely to the next principle.

Think Small

When you seek to develop a new habit, it's important to break the new behavior down into smaller parts and master them one by one. This approach, called *shaping* by psychologists, is responsible for a common truism about habits: without shaping, there's little likelihood of creating a new habit. As an example, think of someone who wants to quit smoking. Examples of shaping might include learning new relaxation strategies, taking a short walk after eating in lieu of smoking, phasing out smoking at night, or decreasing the number of smoking breaks with coworkers. All of these behaviors may eventually be important if the person is to become a nonsmoker, but they must first be learned separately. Then they can be chained together for success in becoming a nonsmoker.

Similarly, coping with daily hassles more successfully requires that you chain together different habits that will collectively have a strong positive effect. For example, if your household duties take up too much time, you might have to practice new skills, such as reorganizing your work flow, detaching from perfectionistic beliefs, asking other household members to help, and so forth. Since daily hassles are a lifelong companion, there isn't an urgent need to do everything differently all at once. In fact, trying to do that will probably just create more stress! Just practice building a strong foundation of new coping skills, one by one.

Accumulate Positives

New behaviors are easier to learn if you receive a lot of positive reinforcement and feel rewarded for performing them. Because of this, it's important to frame your coping behaviors in positive terms. Tell yourself that these are positive behaviors that you're going to practice, rather than casting them as attempts to stop negative behaviors. For example, if wasting time is a daily hassle for you, you might be inclined to define your goal as "Stop wasting time!" However, this approach—focusing on stopping a negative behavior—creates a negative mind-set. If you tell yourself to stop wasting time, you'll end up wasting a lot of time trying to get yourself to comply with that instruction.

A much better strategy for forming a new habit is to frame the habit as something you're going to do (rather than not do), for example, "I will sit down for a few minutes and make a list of my priorities for the next hour." This is something specific you can do, and when you do it, it will feel like a positive behavior. And you'll have something to show for it. That provides positive reinforcement for the new behavior, which will motivate you to repeat it in the future.

Exercise: Creating a Daily Hassles Coping Plan

Your coping plan should include the day of the week and time of day you typically encounter certain hassles and the behavior you'll practice at those times. Be as specific as possible in describing what you intend to do so you'll form a strong behavioral intention, as this is an important ingredient of acting mindfully. You might have to practice a new behavior for a week or two to begin to get a feel for how well it works to offset the impact of daily stress. Once you have some experience under your belt, rate how well the response plan is working.

You'll find a downloadable worksheet you can use for this exercise at http://www.newharbinger.com/31274. Alternatively, you can create a similar form, perhaps in your journal for this book, using the four columns in the downloadable worksheet: "Day of week and time" on the left, then "Daily hassle," then "Hassle response plan," and finally

"Plan impact" on the right. For "Plan impact," rate how effective each response plan is using a scale of 1 to 5, where 1 is just a bit helpful and 5 is very helpful. Higher ratings indicate greater success, while lower ratings indicate that you may need to devote more mindful attention to a particular stressor or response plan. Alternatively, a lower rating may indicate that a different response plan might work better for that particular hassle.

Review and rate your response plans regularly. This will prevent you from continuing to use strategies that are ineffective or have outlived their usefulness. It's common for the effectiveness of strategies to wax and wane, and of course it's also common for life circumstances to change. Developing a daily hassles coping plan on an ongoing basis will help ensure that your approach is suited to your current circumstances.

Gentle Reminders

In this chapter, you've taken the first mindful step toward developing a sustainable lifestyle approach to transcending daily stress. You've identified your daily hassles and rated their impact, and you've done the same with behaviors you use to right the ship and recharge your batteries. Just knowing what your personal hassles and helpers are can be enormously useful in plotting a new course. An important principle for addressing daily stress is to focus your energy on the things you can change, and to work on accepting the things you can't. It's also important to take a systematic approach to changing your lifestyle, focusing on a limited number of new strategies at any given time. Our mantra is "Envision the future, start with the present, think small, and accumulate positives!"

The next chapter will help you take a closer look at your self-care routines so you can create a better balance between daily hassles and daily helpers. Taking a thoughtful, deliberate, and flexible approach to your daily routines can help you build a foundation that will help you transcend daily stress in areas where you may have less control, including work or school and relationships.

CHAPTER 10

Mindful and Balanced Daily Routines

I get up every morning determined to both change
the world and have one hell of a good time.
Sometimes, this makes planning the day difficult.

—E. B. White

One of the main challenges you'll face in your quest to transcend daily stress is creating a harmonious balance between your daily responsibilities and how you recharge your batteries. To accomplish this important task, you'll need to take a thoughtful, deliberate, and flexible approach to organizing your daily routines. By "thoughtful," we mean carefully considering how your current daily routine is constructed in terms of its emotional tone. By "deliberate," we mean carefully considering each activity from the viewpoint of how important it is in the big scheme of things. And by "flexible," we mean adapting to changing life circumstances by changing aspects of your daily routines while maintaining a healthy balance between work and play.

In this chapter, we'll help you develop and implement mindful daily routines that can insulate you from the nagging effects of daily stress. First, we'll have you complete a self-assessment to determine your current balance among daily duties, socially prescribed tasks, and activities that promote relaxation, self-growth, or just having fun. When stress gets the best of you, it may be because duties and socially prescribed tasks are dominating your daily routine, leaving little time for you to take of yourself.

Next, you'll use the information generated in that assessment to help you arrange your daily routines so you have more time to take care of yourself. We'll also help you examine your motives for performing duties and socially prescribed tasks. Sometimes, simply keeping your motivation for tasks in mind can help decrease the stress level associated with those tasks. Finally, we'll describe some daily lifestyle practices that can go a long way toward creating a positive, stress-transcending state of mind, even in the midst of daily stress.

The Power Tactics of Self-Care

One of the hardest things to do within the fast pace of modern living is treating yourself with the love and kindness you deserve. We live in a "duty first" society in which relaxation, leisure, and self-care are things you have to earn by performing all kinds of daily duties first. Then, if you have any time or energy left over, you can do something fun or relaxing. The problem is, most people never get to the end of their to-do list. If this keeps happening over the long haul, you don't get a chance to recharge your batteries, making you more susceptible to chronic stress. Worse, when people are stressed-out on an ongoing basis, their brain functions become less efficient, making it take longer to complete routine daily tasks!

To make this more concrete, let's take a look at an example. If you're parenting children at the end of your workday, the duty roster might call for helping the kids do homework, cooking dinner, doing the dishes, helping the kids take baths and get ready for bed, reading a bedtime story, and staying attentive to your kids until they're asleep. Then, and only then, might you get fifteen minutes of "me time." But chances are, even then you'll feel the call of duty. Perhaps there are e-mails to read and respond to, laundry to be folded, a thank-you note to be written, bills to be paid, and on and on.

When you find yourself overextended, it's likely that the first thing to go is the "me time" part of your daily routine. This is one of the great paradoxes in how people cope with daily stress: at the time when you most need to carve out time to relax and soothe yourself, you're least likely to do it!

Balancing Duties and Self-Care Activities

The task of building a harmonious daily routine starts with being able to discriminate between activities that you truly must perform, activities that you've been socially conditioned to perform, and activities that give you a sense of personal balance. Unfortunately, most of us have been conditioned to automatically perform the same tasks day in, day out, believing that these tasks are somehow essential if we are to be in control of our lives. The problem is, the list of such activities is seemingly endless, and trying to do all of them will suck up your time and energy.

The first step in combating this destructive, stress-related process is to identify all of the activities in your basic daily routines and consider the feeling tone of each one. There are a number of advantages to doing this, the main one being that it helps you bring awareness to all of your activities, even those you don't necessarily like to do. This tends to prevent zoning out and performing entire sets of daily tasks without being aware of what you're doing or having a sense of participating in your life.

In addition, the practice of describing your emotions as you engage in actions creates more self-awareness in a general sense. While you might be aware of the things you really love to do or hate to do in your current routines, it's likely that you're less in touch with activities that lie in the middle of the spectrum—those that are neutral, or just mildly annoying or mildly pleasant. These are what we call "fifty-fifty activities." Depending upon the meaning you attach to them, they can become a source of stress or a source of relaxation and revitalization. We want you to take ownership of as many of these activities as possible and put them in the relaxation column. This is much more likely to occur if you connect with positive motives for performing these activities in the first place.

Exercise: Assessing Have-To, Ought-To, and Want-To Activities

In this self-assessment, you'll break your current daily routines down into three simple categories: have-to, ought-to, and want-to.

A *have-to* is a requirement of daily living *today*, such as getting dressed, showering, showing up for work, cooking, or taking your kids to school. If you consistently fail to accomplish have-to activities, you're likely to experience major negative consequences.

An *ought-to* is an activity that you might feel guilty about if you didn't do it, but isn't a basic requirement of daily living. Many of the daily hassles you identified in the previous chapter probably fit into this category. This category covers things like calling a friend or parent, washing your car, attending all of your child's soccer practices, or pulling weeds. The distinctive feature of an ought-to is that it's something you've been trained to believe is required of you; but in reality, it's optional.

A *want-to* is an activity that you'd like to engage in. These activities often produce a sense of relaxation, enjoyment, and well-being. Most of the daily helpers you identified in the previous chapter probably meet the definition of "want-to." These activities might include exercising, going to a movie with your partner, doing a hobby or craft at home, or going out with friends. You do these activities because you get enjoyment or a sense of fulfillment from them, and that's the only justification you need. In our society, this is usually seen as bordering on pure selfishness. But when it comes to protecting your physical and mental health from the mindless, frenetic pace of modern living, we encourage you to be as selfish as possible!

This exercise might take some time because you'll need to study your daily routines closely for a while and begin to catalog them. To help you complete this self-assessment, we want you to go back to the daily hassles and daily helpers exercises you completed in the previous chapter. Review the lists you generated and think carefully about how often each hassle or helper shows up in your daily routine. For hassles that occur with some frequency, try to determine whether they are have-to or ought-to behaviors. For daily helpers, identify those that help build positive emotions. For the purposes of this exercise, also identify activities that tend to make you more mindful and deliberate.

Next, make separate lists of your common have-to, ought-to, and want-to behaviors and, for each, indicate how often you engage in that activity each day or week. You'll find a downloadable worksheet you can use for this exercise at http://www.newharbinger.com/31274 (see the back of this book for instructions on how to access it). Alternatively, you can create a similar form, perhaps in your journal for this book, using the seven columns in the downloadable worksheet: "Have-to," "How often," "Ought-to," "How often," "Want-to," one last "How often," and, finally, "Activities that foster mindfulness." Once you've completed this exercise, look at the number of entries in each column. Does the have-to column have a bunch of entries, whereas the want-to column has very few? This is what a lifestyle that's out of balance and susceptible to stress looks like on paper!

The Stress Buster's Secret: Shift to the Right!

In general, if you're being dominated by daily stress, when you complete the previous exercise you'll notice that the number of entries steadily decreases as you move to the right of the worksheet. You've probably identified a lot of have-to activities, quite a few ought-to activities, relatively few want-to activities, and even fewer activities that create mindful awareness. The goal of the lifestyle planning in part 3 of this book is to shift everything toward the right side of the ledger!

For example, there might be some have-to activities on your list that actually aren't required at all; instead, they're optional activities that for one reason or another seem nonnegotiable, such as taking dinner to your aging mother, who's living alone and can no longer cook. You might be motivated to do this because you genuinely believe you want to be there for your mother as payback for everything she's done for you. Spending quality time with your mother might be an important want-to as you continue to develop your lifelong relationship. Alternatively, you might be motivated out of guilt that you are somehow failing in your duties as a family member even though you don't feel all that close to your mother. Or you might do it to avoid having your mother call and complain that you never visit. Thus, depending upon your attitude, the same activity can be either a hassle (have-to) or a helper (want-to).

A similar situation exists with many ought-to activities. Depending on your point of view, they can be either indicators that you're living by your principles or simply additional duties you have to perform. For example, while trying to spend quality time with your children sounds like a good idea, there are times when that works and times when it doesn't. If you're feeling feverish and nauseous, you're probably going to struggle with that task. If you have a work assignment or a college exam that requires you to stay focused and work late, it's unlikely that you're going to spend much quality time with your children. That isn't the end of the world, but restless mind will try to make it feel that way, telling you, *You're a selfish person and a neglectful parent, and you're hurting your children.* Buying into these messages robs you of the flexibility you need to address the changing demands of daily life.

Don't Shift to the Left!

Alternatively, you might find that something you used to enjoy becomes an ought-to or have-to. Remember, you want to move the emotional impact of your daily activities to the right, not the left! As an example, let's examine how this might play out with a plan to engage in regular exercise. At first, you truly enjoy the time you spend exercising because it allows you to immerse yourself in the moment and make contact with your body in a way that's grounding and helps relieve stress. Then, without being aware of it, you start to get increasingly obsessed with sculpting your body so that you look good, and with training to such an extent that others never see signs that you're tired. Over time, you keep adding exercise periods and become less flexible about how and when you exercise. If you miss a training session, you feel guilty because you're falling behind on your goal of getting in perfect shape and worry that other people will notice. Eventually, exercising is no longer about being in the moment with your body and moving; it's about looking good or being in better shape than others.

This is how restless mind converts something that started as a want-to into a have-to, and it's remarkably common in everyday life because restless mind always wants to compare how you are to how you could be, and to compare your performance to that of others. When you notice your mind doing this, practice the half-knowing smile from chapter 7. You know what your mind is up to, and you can detach from those insidious messages!

Cultivating Quiet Mind Every Day

In chapter 9, we offered some guidance on how you can behave your way into a mindful, stress-resistant lifestyle, with a focus on activities in your typical day-to-day routine. You could think of this approach as laying the foundation for living mindfully, and the short-term impact of doing this can be amazing. A complementary strategy for creating a stress-resistant lifestyle involves a top-down approach that turns off the primitive mind (the limbic system) and its narrow focus on negative information. A top-down approach involves engaging in daily practices designed to cultivate specific, positive states of mind. This activates the PNS and strengthens neural circuitry in areas of the brain responsible for producing quiet mind. Many of the exercises in part 2 of the book help produce this state of mind. Here, we'll give you a few more techniques to add to your repertoire.

Practice: At the Point of Awakening

The moment of awakening every morning is a golden opportunity to practice quiet mind. Usually your senses and restless mind aren't fully awakened, so you haven't accumulated a lot of mental clutter to cloud your clear view of things. Practicing the following simple quiet mind strategy at that time will help you activate and strengthen neural circuitry that creates both focused attention and clear intention.

Upon awakening, take five minutes to see if you can hold on to this clear state of mind just a little longer. See if you can visualize moving through your day with a harmonious and compassionate state of mind. Is there someone or some life situation that you can approach differently? Visualize detaching from the mental clutter of negative emotions such as resentment, anger, and envy. Envision detaching from evaluations about being treated fairly or unfairly, being understood or misunderstood, or feeling entitled to a good outcome in life that day.

Practice: Open Out

Here's an alternative to the previous practice. (Or, if you have the time or inclination, you can combine the two.) In this practice, the focus is on setting an intention to open to new experiences. Again, practice this technique when you first wake up, before your mind has begun to accumulate daily mental clutter.

Upon awakening, take five minutes to set an intention to expand yourself and your experience. What can you welcome into your inner world today? Can you expand the edges of your personal boundaries just a bit, almost as though you're a soap bubble? Visualize yourself as a soap bubble making contact with another soap bubble—some type of new experience. Can you allow the two bubbles to merge into one? Can you see yourself expanding to encompass some new type of experience and having it become part of you? It could be something as simple as trying a type of ethnic food that you've always steered away from for fear of it being different or distasteful. Whatever it is, vow to say yes to one opportunity to expand yourself, however small it may be. The magnitude doesn't matter; what's important is the act of opening yourself to new experience.

Practice: Cultivating Your State of Mind

Cultivating a positive mind-set is a very important aspect of any plan for transcending stress. People often use the term "attitude" to describe a state of mind. If you say you have a bad attitude, you're really saying that you're focusing your attention on the negative aspects of your day and ignoring or minimizing the positives. And in fact, daily stress can affect your state of mind in exactly this way, making you tend to remember the negative events of your day and forget or discount the positives so that you see your overall day in a negative light.

For the purposes of this exercise, think about your state of mind by visualizing a matrix. The vertical axis represents the extent to which your state of mind is focused inwardly or outwardly. The horizontal axis represents the extent to which you're under the sway of restless mind (negative) or in a state of quiet mind (positive).

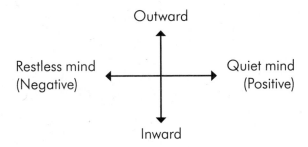

When you look at it this way, at any point in time your state of mind is determined by how much your focus is on yourself versus the world around you, and by how negative or positive your feeling tone is. The result is four basic types of states of mind, as reflected in the lists of associated emotions below.

Restless mind and outward focus	Quiet mind and outward focus
Angry	Amicable
Blaming	Benevolent
Frustrated	Caring
Hostile	Compassionate
Impatient	Connected
Irritable	Empathic
Mistrustful	Humane
Prejudicial	Kind
Righteous	Loving
Skeptical	Passionate
Suspicious	Peaceful
Vengeful	Transcendent
Victimized	Warmhearted

Restless mind and inward focus	Quiet mind and inward focus
Abandoned	Accepting
Afraid	Blissful
Agitated	Calm
Anxious	Detached
Apprehensive	Harmonious
Blue	Mellow
Bored	Nonjudgmental
Guilty	Peaceful
Lonely	Restful
Melancholy	Satisfied
Sad	Self-confident
Self-critical	Serene
Self-doubting	Tranquil
	Unconcerned

Take some time to review the matrix and lists above, then ask yourself this question: "Where would I like to be on a daily basis? What position on the matrix would be most healthy for me and have the best impact on the people closest to me?" Although we aren't mind readers, we do have a pretty good hunch about what your answers to those questions will be, and we want to help you get there!

The best way to cultivate a desirable state of mind is to conduct a scheduled daily review toward the end of your day, perhaps just before going to bed each night. This will help you keep yourself accountable for the state of mind you're cultivating each day. At your scheduled time each day, look at each list and mentally note the emotion words that best describe your predominant state of mind that day. By "predominant," we mean how you mostly felt that day, even if there were moments when you felt differently. (For a downloadable version of the matrix and the lists of associated emotion words that you can keep at hand to facilitate your review, visit http://www.newharbinger .com/31274.)

As you do this practice, try to avoid evaluating or judging yourself; just notice what your predominant states of mind have been. You can then integrate this information into creating intentions to cultivate different states of mind, as in the following practice.

Practice: Shift to the Right Again!

Here we go again, always moving to the right. Since that's what works, let's do it! The solution to ongoing negative states of mind is to deliberately shift yourself to the right-hand side of the matrix. An excellent way to do this is to use the exercise Open Out, just above.

When you wake up in the morning, while your mind is relatively uncluttered and before you shift into a higher gear, visualize a word or two in a part of the matrix where you'd like to be that day. Let's say you choose *transcendent* and *loving*. Take a few moments to affirm this choice, repeating to yourself, "Today, I will practice feeling transcendent and loving." Then take a few minutes to visualize successfully being in that state of mind during specific activities planned for the day—perhaps one for which that state of mind might not come naturally to you due to competing and perhaps negative ingrained responses to that activity. Remember, practicing visualization activates higher-order brain circuitry, which will make you more attentive and intentional as you go through your day.

Practice: Burning Off Excess Energy

The stress-producing aspects of daily life are rarely solved by fighting, freezing, or fleeing, but those are the reactions your body is preparing you for when you confront daily stress. This tends to leave your nervous system with a problem: it's providing the neurochemicals needed to help you physically cope with the situation, but the situation probably requires mental problem solving, not a physical reaction, so you're left with excess energy. When this happens on a day in, day out basis, your body is unable to rid itself of the harmful neuropeptides released by your endocrine system when you're under stress. Because buildup of these neurochemicals can have enormous negative impacts on health and emotional well-being, it's important to develop daily routines that help you shed excess energy generated in response to stress.

Many dynamic forms of exercise will do the trick, including aerobic activities, body sculpting, Pilates, or different forms of yoga. The general rule is that any form of exercise or stretching that causes you to sweat even mildly is probably elevating your heart rate high enough to cause the release of endorphins into your bloodstream. (Endorphins are neuropeptides that chemically neutralize both cortisol and norepinephrine, the two stress-related neurochemicals that are most damaging to your mood state and also pose a direct cardiovascular health risk.)

We personally like to engage in dynamic stretching. It's a great way to use the increased blood flow associated with SNS activation to improve the health and flexibility of your muscles. You could set a goal to learn a few yoga exercises to relieve stress, or you may just want to use your intuition to guide you in stretching. Whatever approach you take, we recommend developing a stretching routine that feels good and creates a mental state of letting go. Associate stretching breaks with your daily activities. For example, you might stretch after sitting at your desk for an hour or after driving home from work. Try not to attach to your mind's evaluations of how others might be reacting. If you practice detachment while stretching, maybe you'll start a quiet mind chain reaction in the room!

Gentle Reminders

In this chapter, you've taken some important steps toward developing a mindful, stress-transcending lifestyle. Although you can't control stress-related emotions, you do have complete control over the actions you take to counterbalance stress. We encourage you to make a commitment to take better care of yourself, even—or especially—during your most stressful times. Building a stress-resistant lifestyle involves balancing duties (have-tos), perceived obligations (ought-tos), and relaxing, rewarding, growth-producing daily activities (want-tos). Another avenue for achieving better balance is to engage in daily practices that foster quiet mind. All of these approaches will help you train your mind to trigger the brain's natural uplifting mechanisms.

In the next chapter, we'll help you apply these same principles to the complicated task of training your brain to take a mindful approach to work. Given how many hours most people spend in work contexts and how stress-provoking work environments can be, this is likely to be a crucial element in your plan for a stress-transcending lifestyle.

CHAPTER 11

The Peaceful and Powerful Worker

The trouble with the rat race is that, even if you win, you're still a rat.

—Lily Tomlin

In our culture, most people spend more time at work or school than in any other activity in life, except perhaps sleeping. (For the purposes of this chapter, our definition of "work" is broad and includes school, homemaking, and volunteer activities; so anytime you read the word "work," please keep this in mind.) Not surprisingly, work is also a key driver of daily stress, and it's well established that finding a harmonious balance between work and other personal pursuits is essential for personal health and well-being (Sonnentag, 2012).

There's a lot of pressure riding on work. After all, it's how you support yourself and keep your family clothed and fed, and it also allows you to buy the "good things in life," climb the ladder of personal ambition, and gain validation for being smart, productive, and perhaps even powerful or a "difference maker." There's nothing inherently wrong with any of these motives; most of them are beneficial to both your own well-being and the well-being of others. But problems arise when people view these motives not as want-tos, but as have-tos. Of course, some of them, such as feeding and clothing yourself and your family, are have-tos, but many of the others are not. To the extent that have-tos start to prevail in your work life, a career you once felt passionate about can morph into yet another major source of stress. This is a trap that many people fall into: relating to work not as a want-to, but as a have-to.

Unless you work in a vacuum, it's likely that you experience stressful interpersonal dynamics or unrealistically high productivity standards. Given how much time people spend at work or school, it's critical to develop skills for being a peaceful, powerful worker. This involves building daily routines that offset negative work experiences and maximize your sense of joy in making your contribution, whatever it might be.

This chapter will help you broaden your horizons and create a lifestyle that balances your work and personal life. First, we'll examine sources of work stress to help you identify your own work-related stressors. We'll also offer some new brain training strategies that will help you practice mindfulness at work. Then, before we wrap up, we'll encourage you to broaden your definition of work so this area of life can become richer and more meaningful for you.

Sources of Work Stress

Each person faces a unique set of work-related stressors. Therefore, one of the first tasks in developing a mindful approach to work is understanding your own sources of stress. To give you an idea of the range and variety of work stresses, we'll share some of the most common complaints we hear from stressed-out students and workers.

One of the scariest aspects of work is that there are so many kinds of "failure" that you have absolutely no control over, such as repeatedly being passed over for a promotion, being laid off after years of being a loyal worker, not being able to land a job after months of looking, having to take a job where you're underpaid, or not getting accepted into a particular vocational program because of cuts in funding. These kinds of uncontrollable outcomes produce enormous stress reactions that can leave you feeling angry, mistreated, misunderstood, and victimized. Compounding the problem, you may take these feelings home with you and work them out on the people who are closest to you.

Even a "normal," fairly unfraught work environment can be a minefield of stress. You might have coworkers who, having invested their lives in their jobs, feel they have no other work options and therefore need to climb the corporate ladder, possibly at your expense. Your fellow students may be in competition with you for a limited number of slots in a program and refuse to share notes with you before an important test. In addition, modern employees are willing to tolerate work conditions that previously would have been considered unacceptable, such as being required to put in lots of unplanned overtime, having work hours cut or changed without notice, alternating between night shifts and day shifts, and not receiving benefits like a pension or retirement plan.

Another major stress-provoking aspect of work is that people often have little control over their work or school environment or how work is done. Most work and educational settings are hierarchically organized, and unless you're at the top of the ladder, there's usually someone above you telling you what your goals are and how to achieve them. We tell our stressed-out clients that modern work settings may be so dicey that it's important to find other, less stressful ways to be of service to others—a topic we'll discuss toward the end of this chapter.

The Five Facets of Mindful Work

The best single approach to transcending work-related stress is to practice the five facets of mindfulness at work on a daily basis. Sometimes people assume that practicing mindfulness is a solo activity to be done alone in their free time. Nothing could be further from the truth! Mindfulness is a highly portable stress management skill that you can use in a myriad of work situations. In this section, we'll show you how each mindfulness skill readily translates into new behaviors on the job or at school.

Observe

In many stressful situations and interactions at work, taking the observer role will pay handsome dividends. Negative interactions at work or school often happen quite quickly and evoke highly reactive behaviors. People get hot under the collar and start in on each other before they have a chance to think things through. From the observer perspective, you can stay out of the fray. Then, instead of being part of the problem, you can become part of the solution. For example, you could say something like, "Do you mind if we step back for just a few moments and take a look at what's happening here? Or maybe we could discuss this further later today?" Comments like this might not always work, but they can establish you as the voice of reason.

Describe

Using your skills in description, you can put objective, useful words to your own feelings and those of others in the midst of work conflicts. If you're involved in a conflict, it will be beneficial to describe your feelings and point of view in an objective, emotionally neutral manner. Inserting inflammatory evaluations into your descriptions will only set others off and drag you deeper into the fray. Describing can also help you mediate conflicts between others, as you help articulate the point of view of a coworker or group of coworkers. You can also become the voice of the group in stressful situations. For example, you might say something like, "I think we're all feeling pressured, and we're having a lot of reactions to that right now. I'm feeling a sense of urgency to meet this deadline, and I'm guessing others are too."

Detach

Detachment is a crucial skill to practice when you're the object of criticism or experience a negative event at work or school. The key is to stay detached from immediate evaluations or predictions, such as *My coworker got this assignment and he is nowhere near as qualified as I am. This isn't right and my supervisor is sabotaging me so I don't eventually take his job.* If you can call on your detachment skills, you're much less likely to react impulsively and say or do something you'll later regret. So describe how you feel at that moment (for example, "I'm disappointed to hear that you aren't going to have me take the lead here") without getting lost in evaluations about the meaning of being passed over. Detachment is also useful if you're being teased or hazed by coworkers or fellow students. When you're detached, you aren't reacting, and your lack of reaction deprives the perpetrators of reinforcement for continuing to tease you.

Love Yourself

If you make a mistake on the job or don't do well on a test, try to remind yourself that you aren't alone in experiencing these types of setbacks. If you don't practice self-compassion when you run into problems, the significance of those problems will be artificially amplified. Extending compassion to yourself will help you put things in their proper perspective so you can move on to the next work task or test. Having the ability to learn from mistakes or setbacks, rather than getting caught up in them, is what's most important in the long run.

Act Mindfully

There's always room for mindful, intentional behavior at work or school. In addition to being highly beneficial for you, it allows you to function as a role model for others. When others are responding to pressure by increasing the pace and, often, the inefficiency of their work, you can model slowing down and taking an intentional approach to the task at hand. You can take a walk at lunch or do some stretching in a break room. You can do a ten-minute meditation practice during a morning break, perhaps using a smartphone app if others want to follow along.

Acting mindfully also includes attending to the balance between work and other life activities that matter to you. If you talk about this, it may benefit others, who are likely to find your perspective on balance intriguing. Coworkers may express the belief that they have to put everything on the line in order to keep their job or get a promotion, an example of the kind of mind-set that increases anxiety and leads to unnecessary mistakes. Once again, you can be the voice of mindfulness and perhaps even lead by example in your workplace. You can invest yourself in your job and do it well, while also knowing that work has its place and must be balanced by other equally important life pursuits.

Strategies for Becoming a Peaceful and Powerful Worker

In this section, we'll outline several strategies for creating a better balance between your work life and personal life. Even if a strategy doesn't fit your natural way of doing things, we encourage you to at least give it a try for a week or two and see what happens. You might be surprised by the results!

Practice: Your Daily Power Pose

Social psychologist Amy Cuddy and her associates at the Harvard Business School have conducted groundbreaking research into the neurological and endocrine impacts of practicing simple nonverbal poses prior to entering a stressful, evaluation-oriented setting, such as the workplace. Amazingly, doing these nonverbal "power poses" for periods as short as just two minutes results in huge reductions in the stress hormone cortisol, with associated increases in testosterone, a hormone associated with confident, assertive behaviors. And in fact, people who briefly practiced power poses prior to an evaluation interview were rated as more confident and assertive by the interviewers (Carney, Cuddy, and Yap 2010).

Before you enter the workplace or a school setting, try practicing the following power pose for just two minutes: Stand with your feet a little wider than shoulder-width apart, with your hands on your hips. Then inhale deeply and slowly for four to five seconds. Don't rush it. You want to get your lungs full without ending up holding your breath. Then exhale slowly, for about six seconds, emptying your lungs completely. Continue breathing in this way as you remain in the pose for two minutes. (If you'd like to learn other power poses, or if this one doesn't work for you, browse the Internet using the term "power poses" to see other options.)

Consider taking your power pose one step further and setting a positive intention for a difficult person or situation that awaits you once you begin your workday. Repeating a little catchphrase like "Be focused, positive, and productive" will set the tone for the day, enhancing your ability to show up, do your best, and roll with the consequences. The more you practice entering your workplace with intention, the more healthy you'll feel on the job.

Power posing may also be helpful during your workday. When you feel stress increasing, lean back in your chair. Open your chest by moving your hands back from work activities in front of your body and rolling your shoulders back. Power poses work in sitting positions too!

Practice: Eyebrows Up!

It is a well-established fact that people form immediate and powerful impressions of others based upon facial expressions (Todorov, Pakrashi, and Oosterhof 2009). The neural circuitry supporting this instantaneous process of "face reading" is located in the amygdala, which is responsible for appraising the emotion tone of external events, such as deciphering the "meaning" of another person's face. Therefore, you're more likely to "win friends and influence people" at work when you're mindful of your facial expression.

In addition, your facial expression is a source of information for *you* about your emotional state. For example, try to furrow your eyebrows as hard as you can and then speak to a friend or your partner in an upbeat tone of voice. Most people discover that they can't do it. When your brow is furrowed, your voice is likely to get lower and your rate of speech slower. If you ask others about their impressions of you during this exercise, they're likely to describe you as very serious sounding, closed off, or even hiding something.

In contrast, keeping your eyebrows in a raised position makes it much easier to adopt an upbeat, positive tone of voice because this eyebrow position communicates both to yourself and to others that you're open, curious, and interested. When you talk to others with your eyebrows raised, they're likely to describe you as friendly, welcoming, or engaged.

So when you're at work and stress increases, consciously practice lifting your head slightly above neutral position, with your eyebrows relaxed or slightly raised. When you do this, you'll notice that it lends a light, airy tone to your mood. The other neat impact of mindfully maintaining this open facial expression is that when you make a point of engaging others with this nonverbal display of curiosity, openness, and interest, they instinctively begin to mimic your expression and thus produce the same emotions within themselves. Then, in turn, you'll harvest even more of the light, airy feeling you've projected into the room.

Have you noticed that when someone you're socializing with begins to laugh in earnest, you start laughing too? This happens because the neural circuitry responsible for producing emotions includes *mirror neurons*—nerve cells that allow us to mentally represent and copy the facial expressions of others. This is the neural basis of empathy: if you can see the emotions someone is displaying and reproduce them in yourself, you can understand how that person is feeling because you're feeling that way too. You can take advantage of this basic neural circuitry by deliberately creating powerful, clear facial expressions that display emotion. If you do this with eyebrows up, you just might create an epidemic of openness, curiosity, and positive mood in your workplace.

Practice: Taking Mindful Breaks

Most people tend to take very short breaks from work and other "productive" activities, or no breaks at all. This is partly due to the problem of overly focused, narrow attention, which generates a driven, negative emotional quality in the realm of daily work or school tasks. As attention narrows, completing the task at hand becomes the only thing that matters, even if it means skipping breaks or lunch.

If you've ever been in this space on the job, you know that it feels like any interruption is a problem. A coworker offering to get you a sandwich is seen as interrupting your work flow, and you're likely to react to a suggestion that you take a break with a retort that you don't need one. Sometimes you might refuse to eat even though you're actually hungry. This is what the autopilot mode of working looks like.

For this practice, adopt a nonnegotiable "workstyle" that includes taking breaks with the express purpose of broadening your attention in order to offset rigid narrowing of focus. You may think you can't spare the time for breaks, but please give it a try. You'll quickly notice that giving yourself a break and a chance to broaden your attention will make you more efficient and productive when you return.

During your mindful breaks, engage in activities that first shift and then broaden your attention. Tune in to aspects of your immediate inner and outer world that have absolutely nothing to do with work.

Because this can be difficult if you stay in your work environment while taking a break, we advise that you leave the work setting entirely if at all possible. For example, you might develop a walking program where you take a quick walk along a different route each day of the week. If walking breaks aren't feasible, you may want to explore guided visualization or meditation applications for your smartphone or computer. There are a variety of applications that offer options of music, visual support, and timed practice. Whatever you do, when you take a break, leave your narrow work focus behind and say hello to the expansive aspects of quiet mind.

Practice: Creating Buffers Between Work and Home

Just as it isn't a good idea to race to bed at night without some type of bedtime relaxation ritual, it isn't a good idea to race home from work or school without some type of stress-buffering activity in between. You need a chance to decompress from the activities of the day and shift from the hard focus required for work or school to the soft focus required to participate in your life at home. Buffering activities can take many forms: exercising at a local gym, taking a walk, practicing a mindfulness technique in your car or on the bus, or engaging in some type of social activity. In fact, a combination of activities spread over the workweek is often best for creating an effective buffer zone.

Take a few minutes to think about activities that could serve as buffers between work and home that you can easily incorporate into your routine. Write your ideas in your journal, then select a few and commit to doing them. It will probably take a couple of weeks for these buffering behaviors to become part of your daily routine, but you can speed the process and ensure success by writing them on a piece of paper and carrying it with you to reinforce your commitment. Alternatively, you can put them into the scheduling program on your smartphone and set alerts to prompt you to transition from work to play.

Practice: Creating No-Work Zones

Most people have heard the saying "Leave work at work." Unfortunately, it's all too easy to violate this sage advice. Work can be emotionally or intellectually consuming, and even if we don't bring it home in our briefcases or backpacks, it can be difficult to not take work home in our heads. With school, the situation is often even worse because school typically involves doing homework, and if you don't do your homework, you don't pass.

We believe that not having a boundary between work or school and personal life is the root cause of much daily stress because it deprives people of the chance to relax. Your mind gets more and more restless, and your body gets more and more agitated by the stress response.

One great way to combat this problem is create one or more no-work zones in your home. These are areas where, by mutual agreement among everyone in the household, no one will study or do work assignments, nor will they talk about work. As a visual reminder, you might modify some classic "no smoking" stop signs to say "no work" and post them in your no-work zones. A fun way to enforce compliance is to have a physical gesture, like extending your arm and wagging your finger back and forth to indicate that someone has slipped into work mode in the no-work zone. You can also set up little routines like doing a few playful dance moves or singing a funny song or verse when entering the area. These kinds of environmental and body cues will support your brain-training efforts.

A Radical Idea: Work Isn't What You Think It Is

We're socially conditioned to take a very narrow view of work. It's something you get paid to do, and the more you get paid, the higher the work's value. This implies that nothing else we do is worth much, regardless of the benefits for family, friends, or the larger community. If this is true, then a stay-at-home parent with three children isn't really contributing anything to the community; a volunteer working in a soup kitchen or hospital isn't contributing; a son who spends five days a week, twenty-four hours a day caring for a parent with dementia isn't contributing; and a person going door-to-door to educate people about an important environmental ballot issue isn't really working.

We'd like you to consider an alternative definition of "work": work is anything you do on a regular basis that allows you to feel like you're being of service and contributing to the community in which you live. Although some of these activities might involve compensation, some are done for different and more powerful reasons, such as helping others who are far more in need than you are. For many people, if not most, the primary motivation for going to work is fear of negative consequences. However, almost everyone who engages in these other forms of work does so for positive, intentional, and altruistic reasons. And even if you have the good fortune to genuinely love the job you get paid for, you'll still find it meaningful to expand your definition of work and engage in more activities that benefit your family or community.

Exercise: Expanding Your Scope of Work

In keeping with the best traditions of meditative and mindfulness practices, we think work for hire is a very small form of contribution to your community relative to other important forms of work. If you situate work stress within this broader definition, the focus shifts from how to survive the impact of your job to how you might widen your work activities to incorporate a wider range of community service.

We often conduct the following imaginal exercise with stressed-out workers to show how work for pay fits in with other ways of making a contribution to the community at large: Imagine that there are four concentric circles, each progressively bigger. In the smallest circle is your work for hire (or attending school). The second circle involves things you do for your children, parents, or siblings—being there for loved ones in times of need. The third circle encompasses contributions to the welfare of others in your community through volunteer activities or participation in community service or religious groups, such as working in a soup kitchen or animal shelter or visiting nursing home residents. The outermost circle includes activities that advance social or political causes that are important to you, such as advocating for initiatives to support community recycling or create a neighborhood park or gardening space.

Take some time to consider each circle of work and, for each, identify activities you currently engage in. List these in your journal. Then, for each, consider the following questions and write your responses in your journal:

- *How do you feel about yourself when you engage in these activities?*

- *Do they have a negative or positive emotional tone?*

- *Would increasing the frequency of any particular activity help counterbalance your job-related stress?*

Also list any additional activities you've been thinking about getting involved in. Consider how you could get started on those activities, and write your intentions in your journal.

If your mind tells you that we're crazy and working for money is what matters most, just notice how automatic and programmed that response feels. If you can allow your paid job to take its rightful place amidst the many other important ways you can contribute to your community, you'll suddenly notice that you can go to work with a half-knowing smile on your face. This is what you do to make money, but it doesn't define your worth as a person. And of course, what you want to be remembered for when you die is assuredly more than what you did on the job.

Gentle Reminders

In this chapter, we encouraged you to view work or school as just one of many activities you do to make a contribution to your family and community. In fact, it's often a lack of participation in activities in the wider circles of work that creates a myopic fixation on the importance of a job or school, leading to a life skewed toward have-tos and ought-tos. You can care about your job without it being the centerpiece of your existence. This will make it easier to lighten your attitude about work and view work-related setbacks in their proper perspective. Plus, taking a new, broader perspective on the relative importance of work-related activities will reduce the stress level associated with those activities.

You can perform well at school or work without sacrificing your health and well-being in the process. All of the strategies outlined in this chapter will be immensely helpful in finding that balance. As a bonus, you might even notice that as you become more mindful and more able to put work in its proper perspective, your coworkers or schoolmates begin to exhibit some of the same attitudes and behaviors. Plus, if you create a healthy, balanced, and sustainable approach to work or school, you'll be in a good position to turn your attention to other areas of life that could benefit from the same type of mindful fix. Most notably, you could begin to bring more mindfulness to bear on how you engage in relationships that matter to you. This is what we intend to help you with in the next, and last, chapter of this book.

CHAPTER 12

Cultivating Mindful Relationships

Love isn't everything; it's the only thing.

—Steven C. Hayes

It's only fitting that the last chapter of this book addresses the area of life that most often puts mindfulness skills (or lack of them!) on display. Relationships with partners, family, friends, and community are so central to our health and well-being that if they are dysfunctional (or missing altogether), we suffer. Most of us have used well-worn clichés that express the importance of relationships in our lives: "My friends are like family to me" or "My family means everything to me." Grieving the loss of a relationship or the death of a partner, friend, or child often reveals the depth and intensity of our ability to attach to another person. Not surprisingly, the powerful and often painful emotions these events trigger can tempt us to suppress or avoid those emotions, or to withdraw so we aren't vulnerable to the pain of loss, rejection, or criticism.

Stress researchers have known for at least three decades that the strength of a person's social support network directly influences how stress affects that person (Grzywacz, Butler, and Almeida 2008). A solid network of social support buffers you from the negative mental and health impacts of daily stress. Conversely, if you lack social support, you'll be more susceptible to daily hassles. Why is being connected with others so important for health and well-being? The short answer is that, at heart, we're social creatures. With few exceptions, the highlights of your journey through life will involve bonding with and learning to cooperate with significant others, such as friends, family members, and partners.

In this chapter, we'll share some insights and strategies that can help you develop rich, rewarding, and mindful relationships with others. We'll help broaden your horizons regarding the types of relationships that may be worth cultivating, ranging from the most intimate to relationships based in shared community values. We'll also provide some simple, straightforward relationship practices that will strengthen neural circuits in your brain that allow you to both connect with others and accept their imperfections.

Mindfulness in Relationships

You may be wondering how mindfulness applies to your relationships. That's natural, as people usually think of mindfulness as something to be done alone, with a focus on how they deal with internal experiences. But because relationships are so important, they're a natural target for mindfulness. After all, relationships can also become major stressors if they aren't going well.

Furthermore, relationships tend to push your buttons because they can bring you into direct contact with some of your darkest fears and anxieties: *Do I deserve to be loved? Am I truly worthy of the respect of others? Am I helping or hurting my children? Does my partner really care about me? What if I open up to others and they find me boring and uninteresting?* Because these fears show up when we make ourselves vulnerable to others, it can be very tempting to check out emotionally, withdrawing and focusing on the humdrum tasks of daily existence.

The truth is, the fast pace of modern living gives you a gold-engraved invitation to isolate yourself and insulate yourself from important relationships in your life. If you're always tired, running short on time, and stressed-out, it's easy to justify withdrawing. You can even cite positive reasons for doing so, like *I might blow up at my partner because I'm so stressed-out.* When focused on your own stress, you might tend to take close relationships for granted and just hope that others are doing okay.

Whatever form isolation or withdrawal takes, it does grant a measure of emotional safety. But we would argue that, in the process, you lose the richness and potential for self-growth that relationships offer. Therefore, in this chapter we'll provide guidance in how you can cultivate a mindful approach to relationships, allowing you to be present in interactions with others while acknowledging both the risks and the rewards of doing so.

Exercise: Exploring Your Social Spheres

There are many different types of social relationships that can buffer you from the destructive effects of stress, from intimate relationships to relationships with family members, friends, and casual acquaintances. You can share a bit of yourself in each sector of your social world, keeping in mind that you need to have some time and personal energy left over for the self-care and personal growth activities you need for balance, which you identified in chapter 10. All of these relationships matter to you in different ways, and they all require you to practice different behaviors and occupy different roles. Also, within any given type of relationship, your attachments can range from intense to superficial. For example, you may be extremely close to one brother or sister and have a much more distant relationship with another sibling.

In this exercise, you'll take some time to think about the different sectors of your social world and the key people for you in each sector. You'll find a downloadable worksheet for this exercise at http://www .newharbinger.com/31274 (see the back of this book for instructions on how to access it). Alternatively, you can create a similar form, perhaps in your journal for this book, using the five columns in the downloadable worksheet: "Intimate relationships" on the left, then "Children," then "Parents and siblings," then "Friends," and finally "Casual acquaintances" on the right. In each column, list people who fall into that social sphere and rate the intensity of your relationship with each person using a scale of 1 to 10, where 1 is very superficial and 10 is very intense. Note that even in the sector of casual acquaintances, you could have a very intense relationship with a particular person based upon a shared interest, such as supporting a music venue or funding a youth shelter.

Next, take some time to review your intensity ratings. Are there any people for whom you'd like to increase the intensity rating? Are there people in your life who have a high intensity rating, but that rating is based on a negative or conflict-ridden style of interacting? If you're dissatisfied about a low intensity rating for a particular relationship, is there anything you might be doing to contribute to the problem? What strategies can you think of for advancing that relationship and raising the intensity level just a notch or two over the next couple of weeks or months? We encourage you to write your responses to all of these questions in your journal.

Once you've identified some concrete steps for upping the positive intensity of particular relationships, commit to taking mindful action in that direction. If you enter into a social interaction with any person at any level of connectedness, you can apply the right type of fertilizer to make the relationship flourish.

The Five Facets of Mindful Relationships

The five basic facets of mindfulness can help you cultivate and grow relationships that matter to you. In this section, we'll briefly outline how to convert skills in each area from "inside your skin" to "outside your skin" so you can apply them to interactions with others.

Observe

Practicing being an observer is crucial during powerful relationship moments. In negative moments, such as when you're hurt or angry at your partner or when your children are testing your patience, taking the observer role can keep you from saying or doing something you may later regret. You can also use your observing skills to better understand the emotions or state of mind of others. When you practice observing, you slow down the process of interacting, allowing both you and the other person to become more aware and intentional.

Describe

Just as applying verbal labels to your emotional experiences is helpful for you personally, by describing your emotional state to others you can promote healthy interactions. Others can't read your mind, and they don't necessarily know how you're feeling in the moment— nor do you know all the nuances of how others are feeling. This is why almost every approach to healthy relationships encourages developing skills in this area. In addition to helping you interact with others well, purposeful use of descriptive words can help you regulate your own emotional reactions, again creating opportunities to activate quiet mind and move toward eagle perspective.

Detach

When you attach to your own evaluations of others' motives or intentions for actions that hurt or upset you, you fan the flames of negative emotion and increase the probability that you'll act in ways that are impulsive and self-protective but ultimately self-defeating. For example, if you attach to the thought that your children are deliberately disobeying you to get under your skin, you're likely to engage in behaviors focused on asserting your power as a parent. You might end up yelling at them or grounding them for an excessive period of time to show them that you're in control. By doing so, you lose an opportunity to take a compassionate but firm approach to educating them about their important role in keeping the daily operations of the family running smoothly. Remember to consciously resist the urge to act quickly and instead take a detached stance before you act; this helps you develop more flexibility in choosing your response. Detachment can foster patience, and patience is fundamental to loving others and yourself.

Love Yourself

There's an old saying that what we most dislike in others is often what we dislike in ourselves. Therefore, increasing your ability to love yourself sets the stage for being more compassionate toward others and more forgiving of their shortcomings. Not surprisingly, this dynamic works in both directions: if you practice compassion toward others, it will help you learn how to be more compassionate toward yourself. Instead of buying into restless mind's negative evaluations of others and the powerful negative emotions they produce, practice putting yourself in the other person's shoes.

For example, instead of struggling with your partner about who's right and who's wrong during an disagreement, you could make a conscious choice to adopt your partner's point of view for a few seconds. Maybe there's something legitimate in your partner's viewpoint that you can get your arms around. Maybe your partner is feeling hurt and misunderstood, just like you are. Maybe the problem isn't whatever you're disagreeing about, but rather that you both want to be understood and validated. Ultimately, people resolve disagreements with intimate others, sometimes after days of frosty silence, by getting to a place where who's right and who's wrong doesn't matter anymore.

A good strategy for shortening the length and intensity of these kinds of mindless interpersonal conflicts is to imagine that this moment is the last one you'll share with your partner. Would you want to remember experiencing love and compassion in that moment, or anger and the need to be right? If you want love and compassion, you can make them show up at any time, even if your feelings are hurt. This may be a bit jarring, but it is good brain training and supports letting go and letting grace, as advocated in chapter 9.

Act Mindfully

Cultivating mindful relationships requires that you act in a responsible, deliberate way even when your feelings are hurt. When you show this kind of restraint, the other person is much more likely to take a similar approach. Of course, in the heat of the moment, restraint can be difficult. To cultivate this stance, start by acknowledging that if this relationship meant nothing to you, you wouldn't be having the intense emotional reactions you're having. The emotional pain you're experiencing is a signal that the other person matters to you; the relationship deserves a thoughtful, considerate approach. For example, say you're lying awake at night ruminating about why a close friend didn't talk to you at a social gathering. Remind yourself that you wouldn't be lying awake if the relationship didn't matter to you, and that your goal is to engage in actions that allow you to use the current rift to build an even stronger friendship over time. So instead of telling your friend off, you might disclose that you really value the friendship and that your feelings are hurt, then pause in silence and let your friend's viewpoint emerge.

Daily Strategies for Cultivating Mindful Relationships

In this section, we'll give you some simple brain training exercises with a focus on relationships that you can practice as often as you want. In these approaches, we emphasize the importance of behaviors, since saying or doing something is essential to interacting. Some of these practices may be challenging because they pull you out of yourself and into interactions with people you care about. If you find yourself getting anxious, just notice that this is happening, detach from your fear-provoking thoughts, practice self-compassion for a moment, and then carry on.

Practice: Being Grateful

The opposite of taking others for granted is to consciously slow down and express your appreciation for what they mean to you and what they bring into your life. This may sound sappy. If it does, consider whether you might have been trained to believe that letting others know how important they are puts you in a vulnerable and therefore unacceptable emotional position. Keeping feelings of appreciation to yourself may seem like a good way to protect yourself from being hurt, exploited, or taken advantage of, or you may view expressing gratitude as a sign of personal weakness or dependency. As you try this practice, you can learn a lot about the layers of self-protection you've accumulated over the years. Everyone has at least a bit of this self-protective coating, but you can break through it if you're willing to detach from your anxieties about doing so.

How you practice this is likely to vary depending on the person you're expressing appreciation to. With a spouse or life partner, you might find a random time each day to make eye contact, pause for a moment, and say a few words of appreciation, such as "I really appreciate your ability to make time for the two of us." With a child, you might just slow everything down a bit and say something like "I can't believe how lucky I am to have you in my life. You mean everything to me." With a friend, you might stop chatting and say, "I just want you to know that I treasure our friendship and want to see it grow." With a parent, again at a random moment, you could say something like "I want to tell you how much I appreciate everything that you've done for me, even when it might have been difficult for you."

Practice: What Are Your Enemies Teaching You?

The honest truth is, you don't learn nearly as much about yourself when everything in life is going swimmingly as you do when your plans are disrupted by another person. If you're like most people, you probably have at least one tense, dysfunctional relationship that can really ruin your day if you let it. Perhaps it's a sibling or parent you've had long-term issues with, an ex who continues to splash around in your social pool, or a former friend that you studiously avoid. You might even regard this person as your enemy. Indeed, these kinds of relationship issues may be part of the reason you're reading this book.

In these kinds of relationships, there's a temptation to be righteous and try to prove that how the other person is treating you is wrong and undeserved. You might even be tempted to get even to show the other person how strong you are. However, others are likely to respond with an equivalent amount of negative energy of their own, so you'll remain at an impasse. Most likely, each of you will continue to believe the other is wrong.

To practice an alternative, mindful stance, ask yourself what your interactions with the person are teaching you about yourself, such that you might be grateful to the other person for teaching you this about yourself. Perhaps you're learning how to be patient. Perhaps you're learning how to hold your tongue when you have the impulse to speak harshly. Perhaps you're acknowledging your fear that maybe you *are* wrong and the other person is right. Perhaps you're learning what it takes to step into the shoes of someone you're angry with.

You don't have to end up loving everyone, and everyone isn't going to end up loving you, but you can see challenging relationships as opportunities to accept a gift of learning from people who push your buttons. If you know you'll be in a situation where such a person will be present, plan to use a cue to remind you to activate quiet mind. One of our clients found that writing a single word on each of his palms ("soft" and "eyes," respectively) changed the course of an evening that could have been highly stressful.

Practice: Reach Out and Touch Someone

Stress tends to create a defensive, self-protective response that often includes physical withdrawal; when stressed, people often don't touch others and don't like to be touched by others. Nothing is better for reversing this negative dynamic than engaging in mindful, deliberate touch. The body is hardwired to respond to positive touch by releasing natural opioids in the brain. It feels good to touch and be touched—if you're able to keep your mind out of the way. Unfortunately, this may not be easy, since touch also creates a sense of vulnerability that can trigger the brain's scanning circuitry, putting it on alert for sources of potential danger. Because this circuitry is already sensitized by daily stress, don't be surprised if you feel a little uneasy and anxious at first when you touch someone. Here are a couple of specific strategies that can help you get past this barrier.

Touching Noses

The practice of touching noses is an ancient ritual in the Polynesian cultures of the South Pacific, where it's a sign of being members of the same community. The cool thing about this practice is that it brings you very close to someone without evoking the mixed meaning associated with kissing. For adults, kissing can be the start of a romantic encounter; with other family members, children, and friends, we usually just quickly peck their cheeks. Touching noses is more universal, and also has benefits in that it can take several seconds and involve a lot of immediate eye contact. "Nose kisses" may become a fun part of everyday family greetings. We recommend trying this strategy with your partner or children. Then, when tension between you arises, you can say, "Come here and give me a nose kiss!"

Hugging a Little Longer

Hugging is similar to kissing in that it can take on a variety of social meanings. But a hug can also be a physical gratitude practice. To keep social hugs "appropriate," people tend to just give brief ones in situations like greeting a friend, sibling, or parent. If you hug someone as an expression of gratitude, just a little longer than normal, you create a space that isn't romantic but is connected. That slightly longer hug tells others that they really matter to you and that you're really glad they're around.

When you do this practice, you might notice restless mind interfering and telling you that you've hugged long enough and need to pull away to avoid social criticism. If so, just notice that this is one of the many layers of self-protection you've accumulated, just like everyone else. The more you practice hugging a little longer, the easier it will be to just let your mind do its thing while you do your thing!

Extending a Handshake

Shaking hands is another social custom that's usually done automatically, yet it is a relationship behavior and an acceptable avenue for touch. Therefore, another easy way to slow things down and show up for a moment of gratitude for someone is to extend a handshake a few seconds longer than normal. Done mindfully, a handshake can signal real friendship and a sense of joy in being with that person. If you're greeting a good friend, you can deliberately make eye contact, maintain the handshake for a few seconds longer than usual, and say, "It's really good to see you!"

Practice: Rolling with Change

The only constant in relationships is that they are destined to change over time. For example, if you have children, your relationships with them will change as they grow. The themes of the relationships change, what they expect of you changes, and what you expect of them changes. The same holds true with a life partner. What helped you bond in the beginning may become a thorn in your side several years later. What works for an intimate relationship in your twenties won't resemble what sustains it when you're in your seventies. And a similar dynamic also applies to friendships. A bond formed by participating in a shared activity like fishing or organic gardening must change as one or both of you lose interest in the activity or can no longer do it.

Mindfulness practice can greatly enhance your ability to accept change in relationships. It's difficult for people to recognize the necessity of change, and the natural tendency is to recoil from change and try to reverse it. But pushing away change is like putting yourself on the bank of the river of life. You can stand there and cuss out the river for constantly changing course and speed, but meanwhile the river keeps flowing past you. To be engaged in life, you eventually have to get back in the river and let yourself float.

One helpful practice is to notice something that's changed in how you and your partner or a close friend interact—some sort of change you don't particularly like. Then try to find a way to view that change in a more positive light. We aren't asking you to lie about something you don't like, but we do ask that you entertain the possibility that this change is actually a necessary part of the evolution of your relationship. For example, instead of complaining that you aren't having sex with your partner in the same way or as frequently as when you first met, you might notice (and even comment) that your partner seems to be developing new and interesting additional ways of giving and receiving love. Likewise, instead of getting anxious about the fact that your preteen child is developing a bigger interest in the opposite sex than in you, find a way to communicate your appreciation that your child is growing up and opening the door to learning important lessons about relationships.

Practice: Checking In Regularly

We recommend that you set time aside on a regular basis to sit down with your partner, children, family members, and close friends and reflect on how each relationship is working. Often, people only do this if there's a conflict or problem in the relationship. Since this is the only time this type of feedback is given, it creates the impression that things in general aren't going well. You can balance the scales by having "state of the relationship" meetings even when things are going great.

As with most of the practices in this chapter, you'll want to adapt it to different relationships. With a life partner, these meetings can be used for a multitude of purposes, such as resolving recurring disagreements or simply taking some time to enjoy each other. With a child, this might involve talking about the things you really enjoy seeing in your child ("Your coloring is just getting awesome!") and then things you'd like to see your child do better ("Would you mind putting all of your pastels away when you're done?"). The key thing about this strategy is to schedule a regular time for checking in, perhaps weekly or monthly, and not allowing daily routines to get in the way. It's also better if the meeting is scheduled for early in the day so you and the other person will both be fresh and better able to collaboratively solve problems.

Practice: Extending Compassion

There's an old saying that in order to love yourself, you must first love others—imperfections and all. When you're stressed, restless mind tends to attach to themes like being right versus wrong, who's good and who's bad, who's being treated fairly or unfairly, or who's responsible and to blame for some relationship problem.

Practicing compassion allows you to consider that neither of you is wrong. The only way to test this possibility is to take that first step of softening your stance toward the other person. As you expand your ability to soften in this way, you'll probably notice that being right is a lot less important than it used to be. What matters is the relationship, not who "wins" in a particular disagreement. Years from now, this disagreement will probably be a faint, distant memory, and who cares about faint, distant memories?

When you approach others with a stance of compassion and softness, try to lead by stating that this relationship really matters to you. Explain that you realize you might have said some things you didn't mean to say because you were hurt, and that you'd really like to see if there's a way to work out the conflict. You actually enlarge your own mindfulness quotient when you're willing to admit you might be wrong in some ways. This also allows you to practice self-compassion regarding the things that you might have done that didn't reflect your principles.

Gentle Reminders

Because relationships buffer you from the impacts of daily stress, they're a critical area to focus on in developing a lifestyle that helps you transcend stress. Some people can help you gain perspective on yourself and the struggles you're having at work, at home, or in self-care. Others can temper your evaluations of stress and help you be less reactive in your behaviors. But relationships don't build themselves; you must cultivate them by taking a mindful approach to connecting with others, rather than withdrawing and trying to protect yourself from the pain that relationships can inflict. You don't have to like the fact that relationships can be painful; you only have to accept that reality and remind yourself that the alternative—isolation—is far less preferable. Remember, when it comes to relationships, the payoff for brain training is more love in your life. And when you think about it, love isn't everything, it's the only thing!

Conclusion

In this book, we've covered a wide range of topics that have either a direct or indirect bearing on your overall health and well-being. On the one hand, we've examined the many sources of daily stress that are virtually inescapable for most of us: the demands of work, school, relationships, and routine tasks, and all of the related concerns. These stressors, and especially their combined effects, can have a devastating impact on your physical and mental health.

On the other side of the equation, we believe that you have not just the power to cope with all of the stresses in your life but also the ability to grow and develop as a human being amidst those stresses. We genuinely believe that if you continue to train your brain, you can turn around and embrace stress, again and again, rather than trying to avoid, escape, or deny it. You can use your brain to help you steadily grow stronger in both heart and mind.

The neuroscience-based approach we set forth in this book will foster a mindful lifestyle that allows you to transcend stress. The five key facets of mindfulness we outlined are supported by basic neural pathways in the brain, and you can strengthen all of these pathways with continued practice. You now have at your fingertips a wide range of specific mindfulness practices that you can use to train your mind to change your brain so that it's less reactive to stress. Rather than seeing brain training exercises as being isolated and separate from your other routines, we encourage you to integrate them into your daily self-care practices, your work life, and your relationships.

The essential dynamic that will determine your overall level of health and well-being is the extent to which you learn to balance the effects of ongoing daily stress with the positive, health-promoting benefits of mindfulness. This dynamic will continue to be in play for the rest of your life because, well, life itself is stressful. Welcome to the big show!

APPENDIX

Five Facet Mindfulness Questionnaire – Short Form (FFMQ-SF)

Below is a collection of statements about your everyday experience. Using the scale of 1 to 5 below, please indicate, on the line to the left of each statement, how frequently or infrequently you've had each experience in the last month (or other agreed-upon time period). Please answer according to what really reflects your experience, rather than what you think your experience should be. (This assessment is also available for download at http://www.newharbinger.com/31274; see the back of this book for instructions on how to access it.)

1 = never or very rarely true

2 = not often true

3 = sometimes true, sometimes not true

4 = often true

5 = very often or always true

_____ 1. I'm good at finding the words to describe my feelings.

_____ 2. I can easily put my beliefs, opinions, and expectations into words.

_____ 3. I watch my feelings without getting carried away by them.

_____ 4. I tell myself that I shouldn't be feeling the way I'm feeling.

_____ 5. It's hard for me to find the words to describe what I'm thinking.

_____ 6. I pay attention to physical experiences, such as the wind in my hair or the sun on my face.

_____ 7. I make judgments about whether my thoughts are good or bad.

_____ 8. I find it difficult to stay focused on what's happening in the present moment.

_____ 9. When I have distressing thoughts or images, I don't let myself be carried away by them.

_____ 10. Generally, I pay attention to sounds, such as clocks ticking, birds chirping, or cars passing.

_____ 11. When I feel something in my body, it's hard for me to find the right words to describe it.

_____ 12. It seems I am running on automatic without much awareness of what I'm doing.

_____ 13. When I have distressing thoughts or images, I feel calm soon after.

_____ 14. I tell myself I shouldn't be thinking the way I'm thinking.

_____ 15. I notice the smells and aromas of things.

_____ 16. Even when I'm feeling terribly upset, I can find a way to put it into words.

_____ 17. I rush through activities without being really attentive to them.

_____ 18. When I have distressing thoughts or images, I can just notice them without reacting.

_____ 19. I think some of my emotions are bad or inappropriate and I shouldn't feel them.

_____ 20. I notice visual elements in art or nature, such as colors, shapes, textures, or patterns of light and shadow.

_____ 21. When I have distressing thoughts or images, I just notice them and let them go.

_____ 22. I do jobs or tasks automatically without being aware of what I'm doing.

_____ 23. I find myself doing things without paying attention.

_____ 24. I disapprove of myself when I have illogical ideas.

Scoring the FFMQ-SF

(Note: R = reverse-scored item. For your score on these items, subtract your rating from 6. Also, we have slightly revised the names of the categories below to reflect the terms we use in this book.)

Observing: Sum responses to items 6, 10, 15, and 20.

Describing: Sum responses to items 1, 2, 5R, 11R, and 16.

Detaching: Sum responses to items 3, 9, 13, 18, and 21.

Acting mindfully: Sum responses to items 8R, 12R, 17R, 22R, and 23R.

Loving yourself: Sum responses to items 4R, 7R, 14R, 19R, and 24R.

First published in E. Bohlmeijer, P. M. ten Klooster, M. Fledderus, M. Veehof, and R. A. Baer. 2011. "Psychometric Properties of the Five Facet Mindfulness Questionnaire in Depressed Adults and Development of a Short Form." *Assessment* 18:308–320. Used with permission.

References

Adams, C., and M. Leary. 2007. "Promoting Self-Compassionate Attitudes Toward Eating Among Restrictive and Guilty Eaters." *Journal of Social and Clinical Psychology* 26:1120–1144.

American Psychological Association. 2010. *Stress in America: Findings.* Washington, DC: American Psychological Association Press.

Baer, R. 2003. "Mindfulness Training as a Clinical Intervention: A Conceptual and Empirical Review." *Clinical Psychology: Science and Practice* 10:125–143.

Baer, R. A., G. T. Smith, J. Hopkins, J. Krietemeyer, and L. Toney. 2006. "Using Self-Report Assessment Methods to Explore Facets of Mindfulness." *Assessment* 13:27–45.

Baer, R., G. Smith, E. Lykins, D. Button, J. Kreitemeyer, S. Sauer, E. Walsh, and M. Williams. 2008. "Construct Validity of the Five Facet Mindfulness Questionnaire in Meditating and Non-Meditating Samples." *Assessment* 15:329–342.

Bohlmeijer, E., P. M. ten Klooster, M. Fledderus, M. Veehof, and R. A. Baer. 2011. "Psychometric Properties of the Five Facet Mindfulness Questionnaire in Depressed Adults and Development of a Short Form." *Assessment* 18:308–320.

Carlson, R. 1997. *Don't Sweat the Small Stuff...and It's All Small Stuff.* New York: Hyperion Press.

Carney, D., A. Cuddy, and A. Yap. 2010. "Power Posing: Brief Nonverbal Displays Affect Neuroendocrine Levels and Risk Tolerance." *Psychological Science* 21:1363–1368.

CDC (U.S. Centers for Disease Control and Prevention). 2009. *The Power of Prevention: Chronic Disease…the Public Health Challenge of the 21st Century.* http://www.cdc.gov/chronicdisease/pdf/2009-power-of-prevention.pdf. Accessed February 2, 2014.

Dalai Lama. 2002. *Live in a Better Way: Reflections on Truth, Love, and Happiness.* New York: Penguin.

Davidson, R., and S. Begley. 2012. *The Emotional Life of Your Brain: How Its Unique Patterns Affect the Way You Think, Feel, and Live—And How You Can Change Them.* New York: Hudson Street Press.

Doidge, N. 2007. *The Brain That Changes Itself: Stories of Personal Triumph from the Frontiers of Brain Science.* New York: Penguin.

Dunn, B., D. Billotti, V. Murphy, and T. Dalgleish. 2009. "The Consequences of Effortful Emotion Regulation When Processing Distressing Material: A Comparison of Suppression and Acceptance." *Behaviour Research and Therapy* 47:761–773.

Grzywacz, J. G., A. B. Butler, and D. M. Almeida. 2008. "Work, Family, and Health: Work-Family Balance as a Protective Factor Against Stresses of Daily Life." In *The Changing Realities of Work and Family,* edited by A. Marcus-Newhall, D. F. Halpern, and S. J. Tan. Oxford: Blackwell Publishing.

Hamer, M., G. Molloy, and E. Stamatakis. 2008. "Psychological Distress as a Risk Factor for Cardiovascular Events." *Journal of the American College of Cardiology* 52:2156–2162.

Hanson, R. 2011. *Just One Thing: Developing a Buddha Brain One Simple Practice at a Time.* Oakland, CA: New Harbinger.

Hanson, R., and R. Mendius. 2009. *Buddha's Brain: The Practical Neuroscience of Happiness, Love, and Wisdom.* Oakland, CA: New Harbinger.

Hayes, S. C., K. D. Strosahl, and K. G. Wilson. 1999. *Acceptance and Commitment Therapy: An Experiential Approach to Behavior Change.* New York: Guilford Press.

Holm, J., and K. Holroyd. 1992. "The Daily Hassles Scale (Revised): Does It Measure Stress or Symptoms?" *Behavioral Assessment* 14:465–482.

Hölzel, B., J. Carmody, M. Vangel, C. Congleton, S. Yerramsetti, T. Gard, and S. Lazar. 2011. "Mindfulness Practice Leads to Increases in Regional Brain Gray Matter Density." *Psychiatry Research: Neuroimaging* 191:36–43.

Kabat-Zinn, J. 1994. *Wherever You Go, There You Are.* New York: Hyperion.

Kalisch, R., K. Wiech, H. Critchley, B. Seymour, J. O'Doherty, D. Oakley, P. Allen, and R. Dolan, P. 2005. "Anxiety Reduction Through Detachment: Subjective, Physiological, and Neural Effects." *Journal of Cognitive Neuroscience* 17:874–883.

Kanner, A., J. Coyne, C. Schaefer, and R. Lazarus. 1981. "Comparison of Two Modes of Stress Measurement: Daily Hassles and Uplifts Versus Major Life Events." *Journal of Behavioral Medicine* 4:1–39.

Lutz, A., J. Brefczynski-Lewis, T. Johnstone, and R. Davidson. 2008. "Regulation of the Neural Circuitry of Emotion by Compassion Meditation: Effects of Meditative Expertise." *PLoS One* 3:e1897. doi:10.1371/journal.pone.0001897.

Lutz, A., L. Greischar, N. Rawlings, M. Ricard, and R. Davidson. 2004. "Long-Term Meditators Self-Induce High-Amplitude Gamma Synchrony During Mental Practice." *Proceedings of the National Academy of Sciences* 101:16369–16373.

Neff, K. 2009. "The Role of Self-Compassion in Development: A Healthier Way to Relate to Oneself." *Human Development* 52:211–214.

Neff, K., Y. Hsieh, and K. Dejitterat. 2005. "Self-Compassion, Achievement Goals, and Coping with Academic Failure." *Self and Identity* 4:263–287.

Maslow, A. 1964. *Religions, Values, and Peak Experiences.* New York: Penguin.

Ochsner, K., and J. Gross. 2008. "Cognitive Emotion Regulation: Insights from Social Cognitive and Affective Neuroscience." *Current Directions in Psychological Science* 17:153–158.

Piazza, J., S. Charles, M. Sliwinski, J. Mogle, and D. Almeida. 2013. "Affective Reactivity to Daily Stressors and Long-Term Risk of Reporting a Chronic Physical Health Condition." *Annals of Behavioral Medicine* 45:110–120.

Quirk, G., and J. Beer. 2006. "Prefrontal Involvement in the Regulation of

Emotion: Convergence of Rat and Human Studies." *Current Opinion in Neurobiology* 16:723–727.

Saunders, A. 1957. "Quotable Quotes." *Reader's Digest*, January.

Schuyler, B., T. Kral, J. Jacquart, C. Burghy, H. Weng, D. Perlman, D. Bachhuber, and M. Rosenkranz. 2012. "Temporal Dynamics of Emotional Responding: Amygdala Recovery Predicts Emotional Traits." *Social Cognitive and Affective Neuroscience.* doi:10.1093/scan/nss131.

Slagter, H., R. Davidson, and A. Lutz. 2011. "Mental Training as a Tool in the Neuroscientific Study of Brain and Cognitive Plasticity." *Frontiers in Human Neuroscience.* doi:10.3389/fnhum.2011.00017.

Sonnentag, S. 2012. "Psychological Detachment from Work During Leisure Time: The Benefits of Mentally Disengaging from Work." *Current Directions in Psychological Science* 21:114–118.

Strosahl, K., and P. Robinson. 2008. *The Mindfulness and Acceptance Workbook for Depression: Using Acceptance and Commitment Therapy to Move Through Depression and Create a Life Worth Living.* Oakland, CA: New Harbinger.

Tang, Y., Y. Ma, J. Wang, Y. Fan, S. Feng, Q. Lu et al. 2007. "Short-Term Meditation Training Improves Attention and Self-Regulation." *Proceedings of the National Academy of Sciences* 104:17152–17156.

Todorov, A., M. Pakrashi, and N. N. Oosterhof. 2009. "Evaluating Faces on Trustworthiness After Minimal Time Exposure." *Social Cognition* 27:813–833.

Wegner, D., D. Schneider, S. Carter, and T. White. 1987. "Paradoxical Effects of Thought Suppression." *Journal of Personality and Social Psychology* 53:5–13.

Weng, H., A. Fox, A. Shackman, D. Stodola, J. Caldwell, M. Olson, G. Rogers, and R. Davidson. 2013. "Compassion Training Alters Altruism and Neural Responses to Suffering." *Psychological Science* 24:1171–1180.

Kirk D. Strosahl, PhD, is cofounder of acceptance and commitment therapy (ACT), a cognitive behavioral approach that has gained widespread adoption in the mental health and substance abuse communities. Strosahl works as a practicing psychologist at Central Washington Family Medicine, a community health center providing health care to medically underserved patients. He also teaches family medicine physicians in how to use the principles of mindfulness and acceptance in general practice. Strosahl lives in Zillah, WA.

Patricia J. Robinson, PhD, is director of training and program evaluation·at Mountainview Consulting Group, Inc., a firm that assists health care systems with integrating behavioral health services into primary care settings. She is author of *Real Behavior Change in Primary Care,* and coauthor of *The Mindfulness and Acceptance Workbook for Depression.* After exploring primary care psychology as a researcher, she devoted her attention to dissemination in rural America, urban public health departments, and military medical treatment facilities. Robinson lives in Portland, OR.

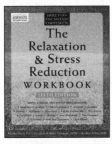
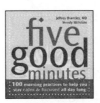
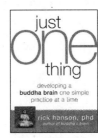
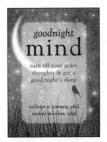
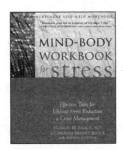
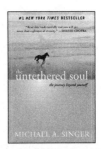

Register your **new harbinger** titles for additional benefits!

When you register your **new harbinger** title—purchased in any format, from any source—you get access to benefits like the following:

- Downloadable accessories like printable worksheets and extra content

- Instructional videos and audio files

- Information about updates, corrections, and new editions

Not every title has accessories, but we're adding new material all the time.

Access free accessories in 3 easy steps:

1. Sign in at NewHarbinger.com (or **register** to create an account).

2. Click on **register a book**. Search for your title and click the **register** button when it appears.

3. Click on the **book cover or title** to go to its details page. Click on **accessories** to view and access files.

That's all there is to it!

If you need help, visit:

NewHarbinger.com/accessories

new harbinger
CELEBRATING
40 YEARS